THE FORMULA FOR BETTER HEALTH

THE FORMULA FOR BETTER HEALTH

How to Save Millions of Lives– Including Your Own

TOM FRIEDEN, MD, MPH

The MIT Press
Cambridge, Massachusetts
London, England

The MIT Press
Massachusetts Institute of Technology
77 Massachusetts Avenue
Cambridge, MA 02139
mitpress.mit.edu

The MIT Press would like to thank the anonymous peer reviewers who provided comments on drafts of this book. The generous work of academic experts is essential for establishing the authority and quality of our publications. We acknowledge with gratitude the contributions of these otherwise uncredited readers.

This book was set in Adobe Garamond Pro by New Best-set Typesetters Ltd. Printed and bound in the United States of America.

Library of Congress Cataloging-in-Publication Data is available.

ISBN: 978-0-262-05096-8

10 9 8 7 6 5 4 3 2

EU Authorised Representative: Easy Access System Europe, Mustamäe tee 50, 10621 Tallinn, Estonia | Email: gpsr.requests@easproject.com

To Jesse and Michael

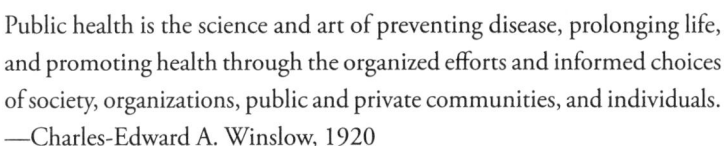

Public health is the science and art of preventing disease, prolonging life, and promoting health through the organized efforts and informed choices of society, organizations, public and private communities, and individuals.
—Charles-Edward A. Winslow, 1920

Contents

PROLOGUE: DISEASE DETECTIVES   *xi*

PART I: SEE

    1   THE INVISIBLE   *3*

    2   WHY WE IGNORE WARNINGS   *21*

    3   THE PATHWAY TO PROGRESS   *35*

PART II: BELIEVE

    4   BELIEVE IN A HEALTHY FUTURE   *59*

PART III: CREATE

    5   ORGANIZATION   *77*

    6   SIMPLE, SCALABLE SOLUTIONS   *95*

    7   COMMUNICATION   *115*

    8   PROGRESS DESPITE OPPOSITION   *131*

PART IV: THE FORMULA IN PRACTICE

    9   THE FORMULA FOR PUBLIC HEALTH   *161*

    10   THE FORMULA FOR YOUR HEALTH   *175*

EPILOGUE: A HEALTHY WORLD   *191*

Acknowledgments   *197*

Appendix 1: Ready-Reference Guide for Community-Wide Action   *201*

Appendix 2: Ready-Reference Guide: Proven Steps to a Long, Healthy Life   *205*

Notes   *209*

Related Reading   *253*

Index   *255*

PROLOGUE: DISEASE DETECTIVES

The black rotary phone rang in my dingy New York City Health Department office. It was 1991, and I had just become a disease detective—an Epidemic Intelligence Service Officer at the Centers for Disease Control and Prevention (CDC). A police detective can solve a murder; a disease detective can save thousands or even millions of lives by solving an epidemiologic mystery. I was on the lookout for a hot lead. Dr. Karen Brudney, an infectious disease specialist known for her no-nonsense approach, was calling to sound an alarm: She suspected drug-resistant tuberculosis was on the rise. If she was right, this was bad news.

Tuberculosis—caused by bacteria that spread when someone with the disease coughs or sneezes—had increased over the previous decade, driven by homelessness, immigration, dismantling of the city's tuberculosis control system, and, most importantly, the HIV epidemic.[1] When bacteria become drug-resistant, medicines stop working and a controllable problem can become a crisis. Outbreaks could overwhelm hospitals; doctors, nurses, and other health care workers could get infected with untreatable strains. Hundreds or thousands of people could die, and caring for infected people could cost hundreds of millions of dollars. At the time, patients with multidrug-resistant tuberculosis needed expensive, toxic, complex treatment, but that treatment often failed.[2] Dr. Brudney's call had me worried, but also puzzled. Did she have an astute hunch, or was this a false alarm? Just as doctors fear the missed diagnosis, such as not finding a patient's cancer before it becomes incurable, disease detectives fear missed early-warning signs, allowing a deadly outbreak to spiral out of control.

To figure out if Dr. Brudney was right, we needed to test every patient's tuberculosis strain in a standardized laboratory. But how? If we pleaded with labs to send specimens, many would undoubtedly ignore or refuse the request. Fortunately, the Health Department has a little-known but hard-won tool, the Health Code, approved by an independent Board of Health. The Code is part holdover from bygone days of widespread quarantine and part essential glue of modern society. It gives the Health Department the authority to prevent health hazards in everything from day-care programs, schools, and pools to restaurants, buildings, and hospitals. Since 1893, New York City's Health Code has required doctors and laboratories to report tuberculosis cases to the Health Department, despite, at that time, howls of opposition and a medical society proposal to strip the department of its powers.[3]

We called several hundred labs and found the seventy-two that worked with tuberculosis. Using the code, we ordered these labs to send all specimens that grew the bacteria in April 1991. Some labs didn't believe they had to, some didn't know how to, and others were too busy because they were inundated with specimens. As I rode the subway around the city to collect samples from the holdout labs, it became clear that some hospitals were dangerously disorganized. Wide-eyed and naïve, I described the chaos to my supervisor, Eleanor Bell, an incisive and dynamic nurse who combined diplomacy, tenacity, and pragmatic action to become the first New York City assistant commissioner for communicable disease. She had created a great team of nurse investigators and cared deeply about the patients they worked to protect. "Oh, yes," she said matter-of-factly, "we call those places pus buckets." It was a prescient comment.

Eventually we had all 518 specimens, each in a long test tube filled with slanted green gel covered by mold-like colonies of bacteria. We packed the tubes into canisters that resembled tennis ball containers and shipped them to the CDC in Atlanta for standardized testing. The results were alarming: One in five patients was spreading multidrug-resistant tuberculosis, a rate that threatened to make tuberculosis untreatable and uncontrollable. Karen Brudney's suspicion was confirmed, with frightening implications for what might happen next.[4]

*　　*　　*

Disease detectives can see the future. With epidemiology, it's possible to predict how many deaths will occur, and from what causes. Until recent years, most impending health disasters were inevitable. Public health had been much like Cassandra, the priestess from Greek mythology who could see the future but was cursed: No one believed her warnings and therefore didn't act to prevent the disasters she predicted. Advances in disease tracking, prediction, prevention, diagnosis, treatment, vaccination, and communication give us new power. This book shows how to break the Cassandra curse and avert foretold tragedies.

Some tragedies don't need to be predicted—they're happening now. In the next twenty-four hours, preventable infections, cancers, heart attacks, and strokes will kill thousands of Americans and tens of thousands of people around the world. In the next hour, 15,000 babies will be born around the world; at least 5,000 of them will grow up with preventable, permanent physical or neurological disability.[5] There's a deadly gap between knowledge about how to live a healthier, longer life and what actually happens. This book shares a formula to close that gap by breaking the Cassandra curse—a formula that can save millions of lives, including yours.

*　　*　　*

While I was in college wondering what to do with my life, my father, a kind, gentle, consummate cardiologist and man of few words, gave me his simple answer: *"You gotta help the people."* This perspective leads to a straightforward question: What will save the most lives? I've been deeply fortunate to have had work that addresses life-and-death challenges and to learn from wonderful mentors, starting with my father.

This isn't a memoir; my experiences and those of many other people help reveal and illustrate a formula to save millions of lives. These pages will take you to an impoverished community in the Mississippi Delta area to solve a mystery, to meetings with angry presidents of the United States and Guinea, to a dark street outside a politician's home in New Delhi, India. You'll hear a life-changing conversation with an epidemiologist who survived a Nazi concentration camp and you'll visit a horrific Ebola treatment unit. You'll meet a doctor who became the first female professor at Harvard and learn about her successes protecting workers' health and the steep costs of the failure to heed her warnings. You'll get to know an incorruptible Indian public health leader, a brilliant and humble Irish doctor knighted for figuring out how to cure tuberculosis, and a cloth merchant who 360 years ago discovered a public health superpower. You'll see laboratories that solved mysteries, others that uncovered dirty tricks of the tobacco industry, and others that killed people. You'll learn about the deadliest mistake made during the COVID pandemic and how to stop today's deadliest pandemic. Most importantly, you'll see how to use the formula to protect yourself and our society.

For more than a decade, I worked to stop tuberculosis, first in New York City, then for five stressful but exhilarating years, in India. Tuberculosis appears throughout this book because it reveals each aspect of the formula. Tuberculosis was once humanity's leading killer. Control required improvements in nutrition and housing; public health interventions such as mandatory reporting and ethical confinement; better diagnosis, treatment, and monitoring; and effective management. Tuberculosis control shows how to see invisible trends, build confidence that progress is possible, and implement simple, effective programs that connect with patients, get political backing, and reach entire communities. In 2002, with the ashes of the World Trade Center still smoldering, I left India and returned to New York City to serve as health commissioner under Mayor Mike Bloomberg. Although we didn't win all our battles, we reduced smoking, improved care of people living with HIV, reduced heart disease and stroke, prevented tens of thousands of premature deaths, and increased life expectancy by three years—a faster increase than the national average. Then, as director of the CDC under President Barack Obama, I dealt with epidemics of influenza, Zika, tobacco use, opiate addiction, and, for many stressful months that almost cost me my job, Ebola. In 2017, I founded Resolve to Save Lives, a nongovernmental global health organization that accelerates action to stop the world's deadliest threats by combining rigorous science with practical solutions. Creating an organization forced me to better understand and explain what decades of experience have taught. Mentors, work, and my own progress and blunders on programs ranging from tuberculosis and Ebola to tobacco control have revealed the formula for how to save lives.

*　　*　　*

The formula sounds simple enough: Expose the invisible, shatter the illusion of inevitability, and act effectively. In a nutshell: *See/Believe/Create*. Success requires seeing disease trends, invisible poisons, and the path to progress; understanding the forces that create the Cassandra curse; and executing a meticulous, step-by-step approach to break it. The pages that follow detail how the formula can stop deadly diseases around the world and how to use the formula to protect your own health.

Chapter 1 shows how to see the invisible, the first part of the formula: *See*. Sometimes what's invisible is an unrecognized trend happening now—as Karen Brudney, an astute clinician, saw with drug-resistant tuberculosis. Sometimes the invisible sends a signal of a future disaster, or of a toxin hiding in our environment. The impact of public health measures can also be invisible; revealing progress or stagnation enables life-saving course corrections. This ability to see the invisible is public health's superpower.

Chapter 2 shows why we ignore warnings, and chapter 3 provides tools to decide which health challenges to take on and how to fight them—to see the pathway to progress. Technical rigor can distinguish simple, effective approaches from simplistic ones. This empowers us to protect and improve not only community-wide health but also our own. Hypertension is a theme in many chapters, both because it's the world's deadliest condition and because effective prevention and control demonstrate how to apply the formula. Similarly, several chapters show how the formula can improve primary health care; such care, which too few people have access to today, saves lives and prevents disability.

Seeing the pathway to health progress isn't enough. When we start something new—a fitness routine, diet, or health program—there's an initial burst of energy. Then momentum can wane and thoughts of failure creep in. "I haven't been able to stick with an exercise program (or diet or smoking cessation) before, so why will this time be different?" Chapter 4 describes how to overcome the presumption of failure—to shatter the illusion of inevitability.

This is the second part of the formula: *Believe*. As I wrote this book, I realized, with horror, that public health's curse is even worse than Cassandra's: Not only are warnings of future catastrophes ignored but past disasters that public health averted also remain invisible. It would be nice if public health got credit, but lack of credit isn't the problem. Progress is fragile. Unless we make past progress visible, old diseases may return with a vengeance. Three strategies help implement the Believe part of the formula: Recognize past accomplishments, make incremental progress, and cultivate optimism.

But seeing and believing aren't enough. Knowing an impending tragedy is preventable is like knowing there's gold somewhere in a mountain—worthless unless we reach it. Chapters 5 through 8 show how to succeed in the hardest part of the formula: *Create*. Chapter 5 shows how to organize effectively and how to strengthen institutions to make and sustain progress. Karen Brudney sounded the alarm for the largest outbreak of multidrug-resistant tuberculosis the United States has ever experienced. Leading tuberculosis experts predicted that it would be impossible to control the disease for at least a decade. I worked for months but made little progress. Then, in 1993, Dr. Karel Styblo, who had spent decades studying tuberculosis and its control, asked me a question—details in chapter 6—that changed my life and reshaped the way I think and work. Styblo's insights showed how to translate scientific knowledge to a program that has saved millions of lives.

Good communication is essential for progress, as chapter 7 illustrates through an analysis of the most deadly failure during the COVID pandemic. But even technically sound, well-managed, well-communicated programs fail without strong political support. Chapter 8 shows how to use strategic approaches to protect people despite resistance to change and the opposition of killer industries.

Chapter 9 shows how to use the formula to prevent pandemics, disability, and premature death. We can see and overcome unacceptable health disparities. You, your children, and your children's children can be safer and healthier. The formula can transform scientific breakthroughs into life-saving programs. Chapter 10 applies the formula to personal health. The chapter uses the See/Believe/Create formula to show which foods, medicines, vitamins, and activities can lead to longer, healthier lives. The epilogue shows how the formula can help create a better health care system and healthier world.

Public health has reduced suffering and disability and extended healthy life for billions of people.[6] Two hundred years ago, no one could have predicted that typhoid, tetanus, trachoma, and other infections would be rare in much of the world and receding in the rest. When Karen Brudney called my office, no one could have predicted that the formula would cut resistant tuberculosis cases by 90 percent in just six years. I predict that the heart attacks and strokes responsible for one of every three deaths today will, if not within my lifetime, then certainly within my children's, be as rare as forgotten killers are today.

To make that prediction come true—to improve personal and public health—we must see the invisible, because what we don't see is killing us.

PART I   SEE

1 THE INVISIBLE

Public health is at its best when it sees, and helps others see, the faces and the lives behind the numbers.
—Bill Foege

Public health can reveal hidden threats, toxins, and trends. In 1991, Dr. Karen Brudney had sounded the alarm about the rise in drug-resistant tuberculosis in New York City. Lab tests confirmed that these deadly strains were widespread. But this didn't answer a crucial question—the next mystery to solve: *What had caused this rapid increase?*

A TUBERCULOSIS MYSTERY

Drug-resistant tuberculosis was killing New Yorkers. If we figured out how it was spreading, we could stop it. Was it the failing treatment system? New, deadlier strains of the ancient bacteria? Or was it circulating in large homeless shelters, such as the one where I provided medical care for mentally ill homeless people, with 800 men sleeping side-by-side on cots in the cavernous hall of a former armory? Tabloid headlines screamed that tuberculosis was spreading on the subway. Fear reduced tourism and prevented hospitals from filling their training programs—medical residents were afraid of infection with untreatable tuberculosis bacteria. New York City, already struggling with the country's largest HIV epidemic, faced the prospect of years fighting deadly tuberculosis.

The DNA of tuberculosis bacteria held the clue. Using genomic finger-printing, scientists can see a world even more granular than what's visible with a microscope. This amazing tool—taking a fingerprint of the bacteria—can show which patients have the same strain and reveal otherwise invisible chains of transmission.

Genomic fingerprinting and other methods to track the spread of infec-tious diseases may seem like recent breakthroughs. In fact, these studies started in the late 1950s, with an ingenious experiment using a technique called phage typing, discussed in chapter 3.[1] In 1991, when we were tackling the outbreak of multidrug-resistant tuberculosis in New York City, it had just become possible to use an enzyme as a molecular scalpel to slice the bacteria's DNA into bits and reveal subtle differences. The technique wasn't easy. Results came in the form of smudged lines on small thick plastic sheets that we had to compare manually, since computerized analysis hadn't been developed. When the CDC completed the lab work on the specimens from April of 1991, I flew from New York City, where CDC had posted me to the Health Department for two years, to CDC headquarters in Atlanta. I spread hundreds of the plastic sheets with blurred lines onto large rutted wooden tables in the antiquated World War II–era hut that housed the tuberculosis laboratory. For three weeks, from early morning to late night, I examined 80,000 pairings and identified thirty-one distinct clusters—outbreaks within the outbreak. Our team then analyzed each cluster to figure out how the patients were connected. We tracked hundreds of patients' movements over prior years and matched exact dates and locations of hospitalizations, jail time, and homeless shelter stays—classic disease detective work. Painstak-ingly, we identified overlaps—dates when infectious tuberculosis patients were in the same place at the same time as people who later developed tuber-culosis with the same strain. Genomic tools don't replace traditional epide-miology; they can make surveillance more accurate, faster, and definitive.

The results were eye-opening. Most patients with multidrug-resistant tuberculosis were part of identifiable clusters, and more than half had been infected in hospitals.[2] The pattern became clear: Vulnerable people, espe-cially those living with HIV, were infected during hospitalizations for other conditions. DNA fingerprinting revealed what had been invisible: Extensive spread within hospitals was the driving force behind New York City's outbreak of multidrug-resistant tuberculosis. Eleanor Bell's insight about "pus bucket" hospitals had been spot-on.

The administrator of St. Clare's Hospital in the Hell's Kitchen neighborhood of New York City managed his hospital with an iron fist. Unsmiling and prickly, he viewed me, the health department, and the CDC as enemies. He had tried to block our investigation, refusing access to medical records, the hospital laboratory, and staff. But, with the authority of the Health Code, medical record by medical record, staff interview by staff interview, specimen by specimen, we put the pieces of the puzzle together. We then met with the administrator and his staff and showed them irrefutable proof—to force him to see what we had suspected and he had denied for months: St. Clare's was a virtual factory for multidrug-resistant tuberculosis. Dozens of patients were infected there with a highly resistant, virulent strain of the bacteria, and nearly all had died. A doctor at the hospital told me that the administrator, who finally saw the fiasco his hospital had caused, drove home that night, put his clothes in a sealed plastic bag, and took a hot shower for an hour, trying to scrub away the contagion.[3]

A few hospitals like St. Clare's (since shuttered) accounted for a large proportion of multidrug-resistant cases. These hospitals had been doing almost everything wrong. They missed the diagnosis of tuberculosis and therefore didn't isolate infectious patients. They ordered the wrong lab tests, ignored results, and treated patients with the wrong medications or the wrong dosages of the right medications. They placed people who had HIV infection without tuberculosis in the same room as patients with untreated, infectious multidrug-resistant tuberculosis. The greatest mystery might have been why there weren't even more cases.

Karen Brudney saw the increase in drug-resistant tuberculosis. Genomic analysis, combined with detailed epidemiologic investigations, solved the mystery of the source of the increase—seeing the invisible in order to control it. But sometimes surveillance can reveal a pattern that's invisible because it is too large, not too small, to see.

Ebola is a scary disease. The virus destroys vital organs, causes uncontrollable bleeding, and can kill half the people it infects. It had previously caused isolated clusters—devastating, but contained within weeks or a few months. Then, in 2014, Ebola hit the three West African countries of Guinea, Liberia, and Sierra Leone, which had never experienced the disease before. Ebola killed doctors, nurses, and other health care workers. Hospitals closed. People were afraid to go to health facilities and therefore died at home of malaria or in childbirth. It was the world's first Ebola epidemic.

Despite—or perhaps because of—their rich deposits of gold, diamonds, and other precious minerals, the three countries faced enormous challenges. Each was devastated by exploitation of natural resources, violence, and the legacy of slavery. Sierra Leone and Liberia had recently emerged from gruesome civil wars; Guinea had just elected a new government after a military coup. All three had weak health systems, and years of conflict left communities with deep distrust of government.

Ebola was spreading fast, and, despite sending hundreds of CDC staff to join the fight and working almost every waking hour, we were falling further behind. It was five years into my time as CDC director, and I felt increasingly frantic. In meeting after meeting, I tried to convince other parts of the US government to do more, faster, but couldn't convey the urgency needed. It felt like another Cassandra moment.

A single graph broke the Cassandra curse. Martin Meltzer, a CDC economist, had developed models to understand influenza and other infectious diseases. Now he created a graph that revealed the potential future trajectory of the Ebola epidemic—to see an otherwise invisible future trend. On calls that lasted past midnight for many days in a row, I grilled Martin on his Ebola model until we were both certain of its accuracy. I shared his results with a dramatic "table drop"—handing out hard copies during a high-level meeting in the Situation Room of the White House. Martin's Ebola model showed in one stunning image that without urgent action, the number of Ebola cases in West Africa could increase in the shape of a hockey stick and exceed one million (figure 1.1).[4]

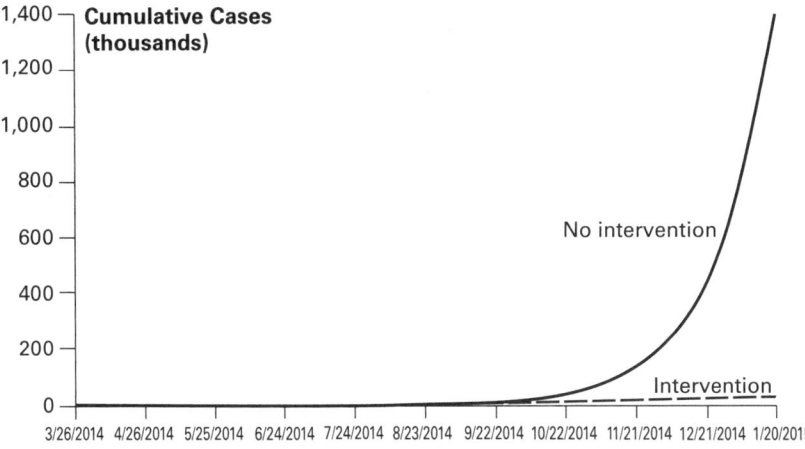

Figure 1.1

Projected cases of Ebola without and with urgent intervention, West Africa, 2014–2015. Martin Meltzer's model showed that rapidly improving care and burial practices would make the difference between control (dashed line) and exponential growth of Ebola (solid line). The chart ends, in a true coincidence, at the time of the State of the Union address. Reproduced from Martin I. Meltzer et al., "Estimating the Future Number of Cases in the Ebola Epidemic–Liberia and Sierra Leone, 2014–2015," *Morbidity and Mortality Weekly Report, Supplement* 63, no. 03 (September 26, 2014).

Martin's model projected that cases would double every three weeks. He also found, surprisingly and usefully, that making care safer for at least 70 percent of the ill and burial safer for at least 70 percent of those dying from Ebola would cause cases to decrease just as abruptly.[5] The graph galvanized US action and accelerated the global and community response that ultimately stopped the Ebola epidemic.[6]

Martin's prediction proved astonishingly accurate. Figure 1.2 shows how closely the shape of the prediction for what would happen if communities implemented effective control measures (solid line) matches what happened in the following months (dotted lines).[7] Martin's model revealed both the previously invisible impending explosion of cases and the pathway to avert it.

Genomic sequencing solved the mystery of how drug-resistant tuberculosis spread in New York City, and Martin Meltzer's projections helped end the deadly Ebola epidemic. But these are only specific examples of a broader concept—one with a surprising history.

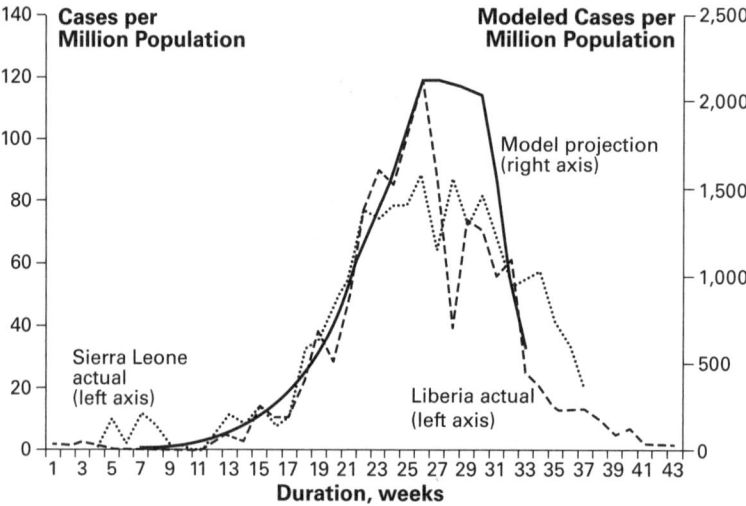

Figure 1.2

Actual cases of Ebola after implementation of control measures, Liberia and Sierra Leone, 2014–2015. The shape of the observed decrease in Ebola cases in Liberia (dashed line) and Sierra Leone (dotted line) closely tracked the Meltzer prediction (solid line). Reproduced from Thomas R. Frieden and Inger K. Damon, "Ebola in West Africa–CDC's Role in Epidemic Detection, Control, and Prevention," *Emerging Infectious Diseases* 21, no. 11 (November 1, 2015): 1897–1905.

A CLOTH MERCHANT'S DISCOVERY

Surveillance, the systematic collection and analysis of health data, gives public health the superpower to see the invisible. Its roots go back centuries. A London cloth merchant discovered this power in 1662, publishing *Natural and Political Observations Made upon the Bills of Mortality*.[8] John Graunt described his booklet as "a new thing"—and it was.

By examining records from more than fifty years of births, deaths, and disease outbreaks in London, Graunt uncovered hidden trends. In different years, plague accounted for between 1 percent and 82 percent of deaths. He revealed that an overall indicator of the health of a society is the proportion of deaths that occur among people over age seventy. (The proportion: 7 percent in his day; 70 percent in the US today; 80 percent in the world's healthiest societies; ideally 100 percent.) He showed that stigma and sloppiness led to the underreporting of certain causes of death. He tracked emerging threats.

Rickets was easy to recognize: fragile, deformed bones, profound weakness, then death. Caused by vitamin D deficiency, rickets increased steadily from 1633 to 1660. Childbirth was fatal in one of every 200 pregnancies—the same rate as in some low-income countries today—and one-third of children died before their sixth birthday. He saw how different diseases shaped the economy differently, noting that plague killed more people but epidemic fever made more people sick, leaving "scarce hands enough to take in" the harvest. And he hypothesized that air pollution from burning coal was deadly. Graunt was a member of the ruling council of London, and this first study of public health data recognized its political implications—something we too often forget, deny, or neglect.

Surveillance sounds scary—like government snooping; monitoring might be a better term. But in public health, surveillance has a specific meaning: *the ongoing, systematic collection, analysis, and interpretation of health information, with dissemination of that information to those who need to know.* Every part of that definition is essential to see the invisible and save lives. A one-time or nonsystematic study can't see trends. In the 1980s, after decades of systematic surveillance, having seen no warning signs and facing budget cuts, the CDC stopped nationwide monitoring of drug-resistant tuberculosis; continued surveillance would have detected the deadly increase years before Karen Brudney did. Data analysis and interpretation are complex skills and if done wrong lead to false conclusions. And without dissemination to those who can act—ranging from the public to presidents—surveillance is useless. Chapter 10 shows how to use this superpower to protect your own life.

Surveillance poses ethical challenges. Dr. Hermann Biggs, who initiated public health surveillance in the United States in 1890, emphasized that reporting health data to authorities is different from making it public.[9] Reporting tuberculosis and other communicable diseases enables support for patients, protective measures for people exposed, and understanding and control of outbreaks. Public health must maintain confidentiality, collect the minimum amount of data needed to protect health, use the information only for public health purposes, and interpret it correctly and responsibly.[10] Surveillance is public health's superpower, but its kryptonite is data breaches and loss of confidentiality, which, fortunately, have been rare.[11]

Disease surveillance, including during outbreak investigations, always starts with a case definition—defining, by person, place, and time, what counts as a case or suspected case. Getting the definition right can be crucial to stop an outbreak. An early error in the response to COVID in the United States limited the case definition to people who had traveled to an area with COVID. By not recognizing the risk of spread within the United States, the case definition delayed recognition and testing by doctors and public health programs and resulted in faster initial spread.[12] Analyzing births and deaths—as Graunt did more than 360 years ago but something still not done in much of the world today—is a crucially important form of surveillance.[13] In 1839, British epidemiologist William Farr wrote, "The death rate is a fact; anything beyond this is an inference."[14]

Surveillance can also reveal hidden differences in disease patterns. In 1991, tuberculosis was ten times more common in Harlem than in wealthy New York City neighborhoods, and the rate in Harlem had been elevated for a decade. Earlier action to stop spread in Harlem would have made the citywide outbreak less severe. Differences by neighborhood, race, ethnicity, sex, economic status, and other factors can identify groups hit hard by preventable disease. HIV among men who have sex with men, opiate overdoses in rural White communities, and hypertension-related deaths among Black Americans can only be addressed effectively by reaching these communities. Black Americans constitute about 14 percent of the US population, but because of higher rates of hypertension and less effective treatment, account for 28 percent of deaths from cardiovascular disease under age sixty-five.[15]

Surveillance doesn't just track tuberculosis, Ebola, other microbes, and trends in births and deaths. Public health's superpower can also reveal invisible forces that harm and kill.

MYSTERY DISEASE

In 2010, early in my time as CDC director, I visited Nigeria to strengthen our collaboration on disease control. Doctors told me of a terrible outbreak. In villages of the Anka area of Zamfara, a state in northern Nigeria, dozens of children and adults died after developing severe abdominal pain, headache, and seizures. It was a tragedy; it was also a mystery.

The most likely cause of an increase in childhood deaths in Africa is malaria, which kills more than 400,000 children a year and can cause seizures. But there was no report of the spiking fevers that characterize malaria. Lack of fever also made pneumonia, the most common cause of childhood death, less likely. The absence of diarrhea and dehydration ruled out cholera and other intestinal infections, the third most common cause of death. Seizures can be a symptom of meningitis, which at the time spread rapidly in the region, but, again, the lack of fever made this unlikely. Infection with the pork tapeworm doesn't cause fever and can cause seizures. The parasite, *Taenia solium*, grows up to thirty feet long in human intestines. If people consume microscopic parasite eggs in contaminated food or water, these eggs hatch in the intestine and larvae can invade the brain, causing a disease known as cysticercosis. This is a common cause of seizures in much of the world. But the Anka region is largely Muslim, so pork exposure was less likely, and, serious as cysticercosis is, it doesn't cause dozens of deaths in one area in a short time.

Investigation found that none of the above caused the sudden increase in deaths. It took time and specialized laboratory testing to conclude something that would have been obvious to public health experts a hundred years ago: The combination of abdominal pain, headaches, seizures, and death is a classic presentation of lead poisoning.

Lead stores energy in batteries, shields against radiation, gives glass crystal its brilliance, and makes paint more luminous and cars run more smoothly. Unfortunately, it's toxic. Lead accumulates in our bones, brains, and other organs. It causes cognitive impairment, hyperactivity, and other behavioral problems in children and is associated with delinquency and violence, lower income, reduced fertility, and increased heart and kidney disease.[16] More than 2,000 years ago, Vitruvius, a Roman architect and engineer, warned against using lead pipes to carry drinking water.[17] Despite his warning, lead poisoning may have contributed to the downfall of the Roman Empire through the use of lead in wine, bowls, cups, and cosmetics.[18] The harms of lead were largely forgotten or invisible until the twentieth century.

In the Anka region, impoverished villagers had taken soil home from abandoned illegal mines to refine it for traces of gold ore. What they didn't know was that the soil was full of lead. Médecins Sans Frontières (MSF) and local public health staff, who learned of the outbreak when tracking meningitis in the area, conducted a detailed investigation. They drew blood from hundreds of children; every child had lead poisoning and in 85 percent, levels were so high they exceeded the limit of their portable machine. Samples flown to the CDC in Atlanta demonstrated extraordinarily high levels—nearly every child urgently needed chelation to reduce the effects of lead poisoning. In the following years, MSF provided chelation to thousands of children and the government and community organizations undertook the complex job of environmental remediation, laying fresh soil over acres of contaminated land to prevent continued poisoning.[19]

The Nigerian incident was one of a series of tragedies that result from the invisibility of lead poisoning. A century earlier, one doctor's pioneering work used the superpower of seeing the invisible to track industry-related lead poisoning. Her studies revealed lead's dangers and protected workers, but government and industry ignored her warnings, with almost unimaginably devastating results.

PREVENTABLE MASS POISONING

Alice Hamilton, an exceptional and tenacious physician born in 1869, created the field of worker health in the United States. She grew up in a cultured family in Fort Wayne, Indiana; her sister Edith became a best-selling author on Greek and Roman thought. Dr. Hamilton joined the social justice advocate Jane Addams's Hull House Settlement in Chicago. There she met a who's who of reformers and intellectuals, including the suffragist Susan B. Anthony, the education reformer John Dewey, the activist Mother Jones, future Supreme Court Justice Felix Frankfurter, prominent socialist Eugene V. Debs, and Upton Sinclair, author of *The Jungle*—a book largely responsible for the first food safety measures in the United States.[20] Support for workers was integral to Hull House, where, Hamilton wrote, "one got into the labor movement as a matter of course, without realizing how or when."[21]

Hamilton used the superpower of surveillance to see past obvious injuries and find invisible toxins. Mangled arms and lost fingers were dramatic but harmed far fewer workers than "the less spectacular hazard of sickness from some industrial poison."[22] She wrote: "Accidents in industry are striking, dramatic, and the cause is clear, while occupational disease comes on slowly and insidiously, and the responsibility [of the companies employing the workers] is more easily evaded."[23]

Hamilton was meticulous. She searched for every case and reviewed every step in industrial production processes to identify how exposures occurred and figure out how to stop them. Challenged by a factory owner who believed that none of his workers had developed lead poisoning, she scoured local hospitals, spoke with social workers, and visited pharmacists. She identified twenty-two workers who had left the factory due to disability from lead poisoning and therefore were invisible to the factory owner. Hamilton advocated for government regulation and organized worker action to reduce risks. When neither regulation nor worker demands were possible, she used astonishing tact to persuade factory owners and managers to implement safety procedures.[24] Hamilton made factory owners see invisible cases and take action to prevent them; the US government would be much harder to convince.

Hamilton investigated and controlled lead poisoning and other hazards in workplaces for decades. In 1919, she became the first woman appointed to the faculty of Harvard University. On October 26, 1924, severe illness struck workers at a Standard Oil Company lab in New Jersey. The lab had been developing processes to add lead to gasoline. Within a week, forty of forty-nine workers were either dead or severely ill. The deaths triggered intense media attention. Despite initial denials from the company, which blamed the illness on alcoholism or other worker behaviors, investigation revealed that the cause was lead poisoning.[25] In the aftermath, hearings investigated the potential risks of adding lead to gasoline.

Based on her meticulous studies of industrial uses of lead, Hamilton argued forcefully against the automobile and gasoline companies' plan to add lead to fuel: "I am not one of those who believe that the use of this leaded gasoline can ever be made safe."[26] She saw that industrial pollutants such as lead weren't just a problem for workers but would seep into the environment—and into people's bodies: "You may control conditions within a factory, but how are you going to control the whole country?"[27] Her colleague Yandell Henderson predicted, with uncanny accuracy, that "conditions would grow worse so gradually and the development of lead poisoning will come on so insidiously . . . that leaded gasoline will be in nearly universal use and large numbers of cars would have been sold . . . before the public and the government awaken to the situation."[28] Gradual worsening is another route to invisibility. Low-level exposures are less visible but can cause much more widespread harm than dramatic cases of lead poisoning.

It's almost impossible to convey the extent of this tragedy. Government ignored Hamilton's warning, and for fifty years lead spewed from every car's tailpipe, contaminating the air, soil, and bodies of generations. By the 1970s, the average American child had a blood lead level higher than what today triggers urgent investigation.[29] Millions grew up less intelligent, more violent, poorer, and more likely to die from heart disease, stroke, and kidney failure.[30] Imagine a country just like the United States in a parallel universe where government heeded Hamilton's 1925 warning and banned lead in gasoline. In the lead-free America, children grow up with their minds and bodies not damaged by this poison. They score five points higher on intelligence tests, earn 5–10 percent more throughout their lives, and live in safer communities. Their health care system faces less chronic disease. The tragedy was self-inflicted. Hamilton showed the danger; government and industry chose profit over public health.

Halting exposure to lead required not only scientific knowledge but also advocacy. France, Belgium, and Austria banned indoor lead paint by 1909.[31] In 1922, the League of Nations called for bans on lead paint indoors, and more than twenty countries did so in the following decades.[32] New York City banned lead in gasoline in 1923—but only for a few years.[33] Because of industry opposition, the United States didn't ban lead in paint until 1978 and in gasoline until the 1990s.[34] Leaded gasoline has now been banned for on-road vehicles in every country in the world.

In recent decades, the United States has made enormous progress reducing lead poisoning. By 2025, fewer than one in 1,000 children had a level of fifteen micrograms per deciliter or more—the *average* level of the 1970s.[35] But there's unfinished business. Now that we see how harmful this invisible toxin is, we must work to eliminate lead paint globally, control lead from batteries and cookware, prevent adulteration of spices and cosmetics with lead, and protect workers and communities.[36]

Hamilton protected workers because she forced factory owners, managers, and governments to see previously invisible occupational exposures, but government couldn't perceive—or was not willing to stop—the broader harm from leaded gasoline. Unfortunately, lead isn't the only invisible and deadly toxin.

POISONS THAT REMAIN INVISIBLE

Although we've made progress preventing lead poisoning, we don't yet have adequate systems to see and control many continuing threats to our health. Other invisible toxins, including tiny soot particles (called PM 2.5) cause millions of heart attacks and cancers globally and 100,000 or more deaths each year in the US.[37] Cancer, neurological diseases such as amyotrophic lateral sclerosis (ALS, Lou Gehrig's disease), Parkinson's disease—which killed my father—and many other health conditions arise mysteriously. More and more young people are dying from colon and stomach cancer; toxins in our environment are likely responsible. Maybe it's chemicals that change the bacterial populations living inside of us. Maybe unrecognized toxins such as nanoparticles are the cause.

Physicist Richard Feynman popularized the idea of manipulating matter at the nano scale (one billionth of a meter) in a 1959 talk, "There's Plenty of Room at the Bottom."[38] Advances in nanotechnology in the 1980s and 1990s led to an explosion of products containing these tiny particles entering the market in the 2000s. Industrial uses, amounts produced, and the range of products made with nanoparticles increased exponentially. Today they're everywhere, from plastics to cosmetics to food packaging to fertilizers and medical devices. They improve tennis racquets and golf balls, solar cells and car tires, water treatment and environmental cleanup. But like victims of the poison the villain uses in the James Bond movie *No Time to Die*, we can absorb some nanoparticles from a single touch or breath. They can then spread throughout our bodies, possibly changing us forever.[39] Despite widespread use of nanoparticles, we know far too little about their long-term health consequences; they may increase the risk of heart attack, stroke, and death. Microplastics may also have harmful health effects.[40]

Other widely used toxins known as endocrine disruptors interfere with the hormonal system, potentially causing cancer, obesity, reproductive problems, and more.[41] These toxins include industrial solvents such as dioxins—dangerous chemicals created as by-products during manufacturing—as well as pesticides and some plastics. The increasing use of these toxins in recent decades may result in extensive health harms.[42] Increasing evidence now indicates that so-called "forever chemicals" such as PFAS (per- and polyfluoroalkyl substances) that persist in our bodies and in the environment increase the risk of a wide range of illnesses.[43] The CDC and other entities monitor some exposure levels, particularly through an extraordinarily important examination survey that for decades has used highly accurate tests to detect chemicals in blood and urine.[44] But this doesn't reduce exposures substantially because the surveillance isn't analyzed in conjunction with long-term illness data, and findings are too rarely used to remove dangerous products from the market and environment.

The 1920s debate about lead in gasoline highlighted a fundamental question: Must public health prove that a substance is harmful, or does industry need to prove it's safe? Hamilton hoped "the day is not far off when we shall take the next step and investigate a new danger in industry before it is put into use."[45] A century later, that day has still not arrived: Companies routinely put chemicals into widespread use without information on safety.

To reduce toxic exposures and balance economic and health priorities, we need data to help others see and act on harmful but invisible toxins. We must monitor not only illnesses but also exposures. We must require laboratory, animal, and epidemiologic research and insist that industries prove new chemicals are safe before selling them to the public.

The final aspect of seeing the invisible exposes uncomfortable truths: Are programs designed to save lives succeeding?

SEEING PROGRESS AND FAILURE

On September 11, 2001, I was traveling in remote West Bengal villages; I had been living and working in India for five years, on loan from the CDC to help control tuberculosis. A small television in the lobby of my spartan hotel showed the second tower of the World Trade Center collapse. I was born in New York City, completed medical and public health training and internal medicine residency there, served as an Epidemic Intelligence Service Officer, and led the tuberculosis control program. Three months later, with the rubble of the World Trade Center still smoldering, Mayor-Elect Mike Bloomberg called to ask me to become health commissioner; it was time to go home.

When I returned from India, I visited my father in his nursing home. During a hike in the Blue Ridge Mountains of Virginia decades earlier while I was in college, Dad had commented, "You seem to like both science and politics. Public health combines those two things. You might enjoy it." I had never heard the term "public health" before. By the time I returned to New York City in 2002, my father's Parkinson's disease had progressed; he was immobile and spoke less and less. I spent hours at his bedside, holding his hand. Telling him of my new role, I said, "Dad, I want to be the best health commissioner." His reply: "How would you know?" These were the last words he ever spoke to me.

Being the best meant saving the most lives, but how could a health department save lives, and how could we know?

In the early 1900s, tuberculosis killed more people than any other cause. By the year 2000, tobacco use had replaced tuberculosis as the leading cause of death. The answer to my father's last question required figuring out how to decrease tobacco use and be certain we had done so.

Trends in tobacco use in New York City were invisible. No surveillance system showed how many people smoked or whether the number was increasing, decreasing, or staying the same. In 2002, Dr. Farzad Mostashari, a brilliant physician epidemiologist, quickly launched what became an annual telephone survey of 10,000 New Yorkers. The survey showed that 22 percent of adults smoked, with no decrease over the past decade.[46] If that trend continued, in the coming decades more than 400,000 New York City smokers would be killed by tobacco and a million more would have disabling heart attacks, strokes, lung disease, and cancer. As epidemiologists, we could foresee these tragedies; we would have to break the Cassandra curse to stop them.

Increasing the tobacco tax is the most effective way to reduce smoking. It was a political fight, but a full-court press by Mayor Bloomberg raised the tobacco tax by $1.42 per pack in 2009. The next year's phone survey documented a substantial decrease in smoking. After another big political fight, we made all restaurants and bars smoke-free, and the following year's survey documented another large decrease in smoking.[47] I assumed we had done enough and anticipated continued large declines, but the next year's phone survey showed that the smoking decrease had stalled.[48] It was scary: We might fail at our top priority. Mostashari's survey showed that we had to reset the program.

The phone survey was our eyes and ears; information on trends shows when programs are invisibly off track. Faced with stalled progress and the prospect of failure, we tried to increase the tobacco tax again, but the state government, which had to approve the increase, wasn't willing. We were stuck. The CDC recommended hard-hitting anti-tobacco advertising at an annual cost of nearly $10 million.[49] I wasn't convinced. That much money is enough to run clinics, support outreach programs, or pay the salaries of 100 staff. Money was tight and it was a high-stakes gamble—would the ads be a waste of money?

We spent the $10 million on advertising and targeted groups with high smoking rates. With robust data from Mostashari's phone survey the next year, we could judge the experiment: The ads worked. The decline in tobacco use resumed and was steeper in groups the ads targeted, such as Hispanic males.[50] Our gamble paid off in fewer smokers and more lives saved. When City Council members criticized us for spending money on advertising, we used survey data to translate the decreased smoking rates into lives saved per dollar spent. If the City Council cut the budget for these ads, more New Yorkers would smoke, develop cancer, heart disease, and other disabling and expensive illnesses, and die young.

One life saved by heroic medical care is a miracle; millions saved by public health are invisible. The superpower of surveillance can make these saved lives visible—but, unfortunately, rarely to the public. The pioneering expert in data analysis and presentation Edward Tufte summarizes this dynamic of focusing on individuals rather than on impact:

> There is a common preference to rescue and extend *named individual lives*, no matter what the cost. Yet comparable investments might save millions of *anonymous statistical lives*, since the cost of extending a statistical life is often small compared to extending a named life.[51]

Surveillance of tobacco use revealed a trend—stalled progress—that would otherwise have been invisible. Using these data, we adjusted the program, helped hundreds of thousands of New Yorkers stop smoking, saved lives, and increased healthy life expectancy. Although tobacco use remains the world's leading preventable cause of death, progress is substantial: In the US, most people who have ever smoked have already quit, and most people who continue to smoke want to quit. Less than 4 percent of high school students in the US smoke cigarettes—the lowest rate ever measured.[52]

Surveillance can keep people safe. Sometimes it's incomplete, biased, delayed, underfunded, or politicized. But without surveillance, we wouldn't have known that tuberculosis was increasing in New York City, becoming increasingly resistant to antibiotics, and spreading in hospitals. Meltzer couldn't have projected Ebola's course in West Africa, and we wouldn't have known if the control strategy was working.

The superpower of surveillance makes progress possible by revealing the invisible: trends within bacteria; disease patterns in communities; toxins; and progress or failure fighting health threats. Seeing the invisible is the first step, but it's not enough. To save the most lives—including your own—we must also see the forces that blind us to risks and block action. Why do we so often fail to see or act on what could kill us?

2 WHY WE IGNORE WARNINGS

People generally see what they look for, and hear what they listen for.
—Harper Lee

The CDC's annual summary is a modern version of John Graunt's analysis from 360 years ago. The 2010 report revealed a troubling trend: US life expectancy had plateaued, with Americans dying much younger than in any other high-income country.[1] Headlines focused on tragic "deaths of despair"—overdose, suicide, and liver disease—but heart disease was the primary reason life expectancy stopped increasing. The trend in heart disease deaths had been visible, but we had failed to act. To save the most lives we need to understand why we often ignore what we see. This chapter dissects six drivers of the Cassandra curse: the prevention paradox, economic interests, the myth of unfettered free will, social norms, false alarms, and hyperbolic discounting—our tendency to shortchange the future. A common theme connects these six drivers: Our perception of ourselves, our world, and our future is inaccurate. When we improve our perception so we see and overcome these barriers (summarized in appendix 1), we can transform knowledge into life-saving action and harness the power of surveillance to save millions of lives—including our own.

PREVENTION PARADOX

The fate of a major initiative to save lives in the United States illustrates the prevention paradox. In the US from 1960 to 2010, a steady decrease in cardiovascular disease (heart attacks and strokes) prevented 20 million deaths and increased life expectancy.[2] Many improvements drove progress: better nutrition, less smoking, cleaner air, new medications to reduce blood pressure and unhealthy lipids, and better treatment of people with heart disease. The lead poisoning epidemic, which appears to also cause heart attacks and strokes, abated.[3] Then the decades-long decline in cardiovascular deaths stalled. Although there is attention, appropriately, to the horrific increase in overdose deaths in the United States, reaching 100,000 annually in recent years, every year in the US, 800,000 people die from heart attack and stroke, including 160,000 younger than age sixty-five.[4]

To address this trend, in 2011, the White House and Department of Health and Human Services launched the Million Hearts initiative. The goal: Prevent one million heart attacks and strokes over five years. We made visible what had been invisible: 10 million heart attacks and strokes would occur in the United States from 2012–2016. Preventing a million of those—just 10 percent—was well within reach. In addition to White House approval, the secretary of health and human services gave strong support and convened weekly tracking meetings. Expansion of insurance coverage through President Obama's Affordable Care Act made faster progress possible. The Centers for Medicare and Medicaid Services, which pays for most health care in the United States, encouraged providers to improve cardiovascular care by using financial incentives and quality measures and jointly managed the initiative with the CDC. The Food and Drug Administration (FDA) and the CDC planned actions to reduce tobacco use and improve nutrition. The agency that oversees more than 9,000 community health centers adopted Million Hearts enthusiastically. The program brought together federal agencies, state governments, clinical consortia, and more than fifty professional and community organizations.

We applied the formula: Make future heart attacks visible (See), convince leaders success is possible (Believe), and take strategic action to drive change (Create). To prevent heart attacks and strokes, the initiative would reduce tobacco use, decrease sodium consumption, and eliminate artificial trans fat from the food supply. For treatment, we would improve blood pressure control.[5]

What happened? Both legs of the Million Hearts campaign—prevention and treatment—failed. Although estimated to have helped prevent 135,000 cardiovascular events, on any test, 13.5 percent is a failing grade.[6] We applied the formula. We made the invisible—the stall in the decrease of heart attacks—visible. We motivated government to act. We had a focused plan. And we failed. I felt frustrated beyond words at the lack of progress on prevention and appalled by my own ignorance about how to improve clinical care. Why did we fail? What had we missed?

We made the deadly trend in heart attacks and strokes visible, but we missed the invisible forces that block progress. Politics—competing priorities, industry opposition, and court challenges—doomed tobacco control and sodium reduction. The FDA, not the CDC, has the authority to regulate nicotine to nonaddictive levels and to reduce sodium intake by setting mandatory targets in packaged and prepared foods. Administrative action and legislation could have reduced exposure to deadly pollution, reduced tobacco consumption, and improved nutrition. I spent years fuming and frustrated by the lack of progress on these initiatives, meeting with leaders at the Department of Health and Human Services regularly and sending strongly—even stridently—worded emails. But I failed to get more strategic because I didn't see the forces that fought against us.

To understand why the community aspects of the Million Hearts initiative failed, it's necessary to understand a cognitive distortion that empowers the political forces that blocked it: the *prevention paradox*. Geoffrey Rose, a profound public health thinker, coined the term. He explained: "A preventive measure that brings large benefits to the community offers little to each participating individual. . . . When many people each receive a little benefit, the total benefit may be large."[7] The reverse is also true: "A large number of people exposed to a small risk may generate many more cases than a small number exposed to a high risk."[8] Paradoxically, threats we can't see kill more people than dramatic disasters, and invisible improvements save more lives than high-profile cures. As Alice Hamilton realized, lead poisoning of workers caused more harm than gruesome, headline-making injuries. Similarly, low but widespread levels of lead exposure, although invisible, cause much more misery than horrific fatal lead-poisoning incidents.

The prevention paradox creates a political challenge: a few powerful entities oppose change, and future benefits that help many more people are less tangible. These substantial benefits may be invisible to each person benefited. In contrast, the immediate costs to a few organizations are obvious and lead them to oppose action. Failure to improve nutrition and reduce tobacco use in the Million Hearts initiative demonstrates the political implications of the prevention paradox: Concentrated costs to the tobacco and food industries led to powerful lobbying, which prevented action that would have had substantial but diffuse and delayed benefits to millions of people. We didn't create the political power needed to counter industry pressure and implement programs that deliver benefits people can't see.

But why did the treatment part of Million Hearts also fail? Improved blood pressure control, the clinical focus of Million Hearts, can save more lives than any other clinical intervention.[9] Before the initiative, control had increased from 32 percent in 2000 to 54 percent in 2014. After the initiative, blood pressure control actually *decreased* to 44 percent.[10] (Pause for a moment to reflect on those numbers. The US spends more than $4 trillion a year—nearly one of every five dollars of our economy—on health care. And we can't get the most important outcome right even half the time. We'll return to this issue.) It's possible control rates would have declined even more without Million Hearts, but that's little comfort, particularly for the people who had preventable heart attacks and strokes.

Could the lower hypertension control rate have been due to the obesity epidemic? Probably not. The decrease in blood pressure control occurred over just a few years, but obesity had increased for many years. Was the problem lack of access to health care? No. Health insurance coverage had increased; nearly 90 percent of people with uncontrolled hypertension have health insurance. Poor health care system performance is the underlying reason for the failure to improve hypertension control.[11] The reason for poor health care system performance illustrates the second driver of the Cassandra curse.

ECONOMIC INCENTIVES

The inescapable conclusion from Million Hearts' failure to improve blood pressure control: It's all about money—the *economic incentives* that structure the health care system. You get what you pay for. In most health care systems in the United States, we pay for visits and procedures. Doctors who take the time and effort to control a patient's blood pressure earn little or no more money, and by preventing a heart attack or stroke, substantially reduce health care system revenue. No doctor intentionally leaves blood pressure uncontrolled so their patient will have a heart attack; the system's economic incentives make this outcome inevitable.

The Kaiser Permanente health care system controls 90 percent of their patients' blood pressure—approximately twice the rate of the rest of the country.[12] Because it both insures and cares for its patients for decades, controlling blood pressure to reduce heart attacks and strokes in the long run makes economic sense. When Kaiser Permanente prevents hospitalizations, it earns money. When it doesn't, costs rise but income doesn't. Patients, doctors, and payers all have the same incentives and work toward the same goal—protecting patients' health and keeping them out of the hospital. In contrast, the economic incentives in most US health care systems pit patients, doctors, and payers against each other in struggles to restrict or increase care.

The failure of Million Hearts and the success of Kaiser Permanente demonstrate how political and economic factors determine health progress. Sometimes the most dangerous health threats aren't microbes, toxins, or trends but lobbyists, investors, and politicians. Alice Hamilton couldn't convince others to ban lead from gasoline for a straightforward although invisible reason: The gasoline industry had secretly paid public health officials.[13] Economic incentives can easily and invisibly block health initiatives. But the next reason we ignore warnings lurks inside each of us.

THE MYTH OF UNFETTERED FREE WILL

When the CDC tobacco laboratory ordered a machine to analyze cigarette smoke, the tobacco industry tried, unsuccessfully, to block the sale. In the years that followed, Dr. Jim Pirkle and his colleagues in the CDC tobacco lab learned why. The details demonstrate that our implicit belief that we have unfettered free will is often misguided.

The tobacco industry placed holes in the sides of cigarette filters. When a person smoked a cigarette, their fingers usually covered the holes and the smoke—along with the toxins—went right into the smoker's lungs. But the smoking machine, used by the tobacco industry to brag about "safer" cigarettes, attached to the cigarette so the holes weren't covered, allowing room air to dilute the cigarette smoke analyzed by the machine.[14] This dilution resulted in measured concentrations of harmful chemicals that were much lower than those experienced by smokers. By blocking the holes, Pirkle and his colleagues made smoking machine results more accurately reflect what happens when people smoke. But that was just the beginning.

Nicotine is the addictive substance in tobacco. Internal documents made public through a lawsuit revealed that tobacco companies referred to the cigarette as a "nicotine delivery device" and acknowledged that it's the nicotine in cigarettes that makes people want to smoke.[15] Although nicotine occurs naturally in tobacco, companies make sure the part farthest from the filter has the most; the first few puffs give a rush of nicotine. "That's why," Pirkle explained, "many smokers stub out the cigarette before it's smoked down to the filter. There's less nicotine at the bottom. The smoker needs to smoke a new cigarette to get more nicotine."

The more Pirkle and his colleagues studied, the more strategies they found that the tobacco industry used to maximize cigarette addictiveness. Increasing the pH of tobacco by spraying it with ammonia, urea, or other alkaline chemicals increased the amount of "free" nicotine—a form of nicotine even more addictive than regular nicotine. Free nicotine is absorbed through the lungs rapidly and goes to the brain in a more active form.[16] Adding sugars to cigarettes neutralizes the harsh taste, encourages adolescents to smoke, and appears to increase addictiveness.[17] Menthol makes cigarettes feel less harsh, reduces cough, and appears to increase the number of nicotine receptors in the brain.[18] With all these features, a puff of a cigarette delivers nicotine to smokers' brains faster than an intravenous injection of nicotine. The tobacco industry ensures there's enough nicotine in every cigarette to keep people addicted.[19] And it's not just cigarettes; Pirkle's lab also documented modifications of chewing tobacco that increase nicotine absorption.[20] Pirkle's smoking machine discovered some of the many ways tobacco companies keep another machine—the human body —smoking.

In 1900, less than 2 percent of adults smoked cigarettes. Tobacco companies changed that. On April 14, 1994, the heads of seven major tobacco companies testified under oath before the US Congress that cigarettes are not addictive.[21] Not only did their companies know cigarettes are addictive, they were engineering cigarettes to become even more so. Tobacco use isn't inevitable; it's the result of specific, purposeful actions by one industry, and every year it kills more than 400,000 people in the US and 8 million people—more than one of every eight deaths—around the world.[22]

When I became New York City health commissioner, I told a newspaper that after a decade fighting the bacteria that causes tuberculosis, my new enemy was a really low life-form: the tobacco executive.[23] Days later, I received a short letter from the world's largest tobacco company, Philip Morris, then headquartered in New York City. The letter complained that my statement was a form of hate speech and inappropriate, since no person should be described as less than human. I had to agree. Since receiving that letter, I've stuck to the facts and refer to tobacco executives as mass murderers. Philip Morris hasn't written again.

In addition to increasing nicotine delivery, the tobacco industry has spent hundreds of billions of dollars on advertising, marketing, and promotion—at least twenty times more than governments spend on tobacco control.[24] (In 1967, a lawsuit and requirement by the Federal Communications Commission gave anti-tobacco ads free airtime alongside tobacco ads. This decreased smoking so much that the tobacco industry stopped television and radio advertising voluntarily, even before the government banned their ads in 1971.[25]) Smokers' "free" choice to smoke is far from free. More than 80 percent of smokers become addicted as teenagers, not as adults making an informed choice. Most smokers want to quit, but smoking in adolescence is associated with lower likelihood of quitting as an adult. Government regulation of tobacco company marketing and manipulation of the addictiveness of cigarettes would increase individual freedom of choice.

We like to think we have complete free will, but we don't. Tobacco addiction is a particularly clear example of the myth of unfettered free will, but that same myth undermines our understanding of eating, exercising, drinking alcohol, and other behaviors. In addition to the prevention paradox and the economic incentives that overrule public health action, the myth of unfettered free will is the third major driver of the Cassandra curse. Rose, who coined the prevention paradox term, also summarized the fallacy that people's behavior is determined by free choice and the implications for public health and for politics:

> We may think that our personal lifestyle represents our own free choice, but that belief is often mistaken. . . . Personal lifestyle is socially conditioned. . . . It makes little sense to expect individuals to behave differently from their peers; it is more appropriate to seek a general change in behavioral norms and in the circumstances which facilitate their adoption. . . . The primary determinants of disease are mainly economic and social, and therefore its remedies must also be economic and social. Medicine and politics cannot and should not be kept apart.[26]

It's hard to see the outside forces that can determine our choices. When we recognize that product design and promotion shapes what we do, we can shift the focus from individual blame to the need to create a healthier environment. But when choices have been made the same way for so long, they seem natural and inevitable, leading to the fourth driver of our blindness to health risks.

SOCIAL NORMS

"If you want to build character," Mayor Bloomberg said, "try banning smoking in bars then marching in a parade on Staten Island. You get a lot of one-finger waves and signs that read 'I Smoke and I Vote!'" Staten Island, the most conservative area of New York City, is politically powerful and has the highest smoking rate in the city.

Making New York City restaurants and bars smoke-free was not just a major political fight, it was also a culture clash. Peter Drucker, the management guru (he said people called him a guru because charlatan was too hard to spell) famously said, "Culture eats strategy for breakfast." Smoky restaurants and bars seemed to be a defining part of New York City culture—a *social norm*. Bar owners called the proposal "ludicrous," and tabloids bemoaned the proposed end of the smoky bar.[27]

Rather than fight against culture, advocates, learning from Alice Hamilton, showed that we could build on the culture of worker safety. We reframed the debate away from freedoms of smokers and bar owners to the freedom of restaurant staff and bartenders to work without exposure to chemicals that could cause cancer and heart attacks.[28] We sent health inspectors into smoky bars to measure pollution levels and showed that levels in these bars were far higher than in places such as traffic tunnels that New Yorkers thought of as filthy. That, along with systematic lobbying and Mayor Bloomberg's willingness to go to the mat, got the law passed.

Racial, ethnic, gender, and geographic disparities in health, education, and economic outcomes have persisted for so long they can seem immutable. Black Americans have a much shorter life expectancy than White Americans, and people in some US counties live, on average, fifteen years shorter lives than people in other counties. These differences are not inevitable. By recognizing them as unacceptable, we can strengthen systematic efforts to change the social and economic forces that sustain them.

Social norms can undermine attempts to avert future catastrophes by making current, unhealthy patterns seem normal. Against this misguided concept of the natural order of things, change seems abnormal. Controversial as New York City's smoke-free law was, by its second anniversary it was a nonissue; smoke-free restaurants and bars had become the new norm. This illustrates the aphorism that "It always seems impossible until it's done."

A generation or two ago, it seemed normal for a family to get into their car, pump leaded gasoline into the tank, ride without seatbelts, drive to a beach to sunbathe with tanning oil, have a few drinks, then drive to a restaurant to smoke and have dinner. These activities increase the risk of cancer, heart attack, stroke, and fatal car crashes. Changes in social norms resulted from health campaigns (use sunblock to prevent cancer; don't drink and drive; avoid secondhand smoke) and, where appropriate, legislation (drunk-driving laws and laws to protect workers from secondhand smoke). Legal changes were enabled by and also catalyzed cultural transformation.

Although avoidable skin cancer, deaths from drunk driving, and heart attacks from exposure to other people's cigarette smoke continue, these are no longer seen as normal, acceptable, or inevitable.

FALSE ALARMS

Another reason people ignore warnings is straightforward: too many *false alarms*. Early warning of an outbreak can save lives—making visible an impending disaster. After the anthrax attacks of 2001, the administration of George W. Bush invested heavily in Project BioWatch.[29] BioWatch placed air monitors in strategic locations in New York City, Washington, DC, and more than a dozen other cities. Designed as sentinels, the monitors sniff the air for traces of deadly microbes. On paper, BioWatch promised to be an advanced, automated early-warning system, but the realities proved more complex.

Years of daily sampling produced false positive results. Some false positives, such as those for the bacteria that causes tularemia, a disease known as rabbit fever, may reflect sporadic presence of these bacteria in the air.[30] The presence of some microbes isn't necessarily a harbinger of an impending outbreak, just as harmful microbes colonize some people but don't cause disease. And BioWatch could miss a deadly outbreak spread by food, water, direct contact between people, or because the sensors aren't where the microbes are.

The theory of BioWatch is sound: If a terrorist released large plumes of anthrax or another dangerous pathogen, the system might identify the attack before people became sick and accelerate the response, saving lives. But against this theoretical benefit is the cost of the program, the small benefit compared with other programs, and the cost of false alarms that drain resources and risk desensitizing responders and the public to true emergencies. In report after dreary report over more than twenty years, the nonpartisan Government Accountability Office criticized BioWatch's waste of hundreds of millions of dollars and generation of false alarms in search of a magical way to detect airborne pathogens.[31]

There's another important, and complicated, cause of false alarms. Figuring out whether a cluster of cases reflects spread of disease or coincidence is hard. When a cluster of cancers occurs in one neighborhood, common exposure seems the likely cause. Imagine three people in the same neighborhood diagnosed with the same rare cancer. If this cancer occurs in one person out of every 100,000 every year, a community of 10,000 people would have about one case every ten years. Three people in the same community getting the same cancer in the same year by chance alone seems highly unlikely. But the US has thousands of small communities. Although the likelihood of three cases of this rare cancer in any one community is low, by chance alone, such a cluster will occur in many communities in the US every year.

The statistics of cluster analysis are complex; the politics are even messier. Faced with tragedies such as the deaths of young children from cancer, it seems heartless to quibble about numbers. And in truth, it's often impossible to determine whether a specific exposure caused a specific cancer. We may never know whether some alarms, such as a cancer cluster, are accurate or false. Understanding that clusters don't prove causality and that alarms may be accurate, false, or indeterminate can help us tolerate false alarms without undermining confidence in warnings of true catastrophes.

HYPERBOLIC DISCOUNTING

The final driver of the curse is *hyperbolic discounting*, which leads us to underestimate—and therefore be more likely to experience—future suffering.[32] It's a complicated but important term. Think of it as shortchanging the future. Doctors see this all the time: I can never forget my sweet, feisty older patient with severe emphysema, and not only because she gave me a huge red tin of cookie wafers. She gasped for every breath and, as she died, expressed deep remorse that she had smoked for so many years. Skipping medication, enjoying a delicious dessert, and lounging instead of exercising provide short-term benefits that may overshadow long-term health consequences. We tend to overestimate the risk of short-term dangers, especially those we feel we can't control—shark attacks, a stranger harming our children, an elevator malfunctioning. We underestimate longer-term risks, such as those from smoking and hypertension, and from those we feel we control, such as driving too fast.[33]

Related to hyperbolic discounting, the normalcy bias, known more evocatively as the ostrich effect, subverts our recognition of risk. People tend to believe that things will continue as they have and to underestimate the likelihood and severity of a disaster. Normalcy bias explains why people often fail to prepare for—and why many people don't respond promptly to—hurricanes, volcanoes, earthquakes, and pandemics.[34]

WHY WE LACK GOOD PRIMARY HEALTH CARE

To see how the drivers of the Cassandra curse combine and how to counteract them, consider our lack of an effective primary health care system, in which clinicians provide ongoing, comprehensive care to address most health care needs. Primary health care works best when a team collaborates to provide high-quality treatment, prevent illness, and find problems early. Good primary care can save individual patients' lives—and transform the health of countries.

In 1950, people in Thailand had a life expectancy twenty-five years shorter than in the United States. By 2019, Thais were living as long as Americans—seventy-nine years. By 2021, they were living a year and a half longer, despite having a much lower per capita income. Costa Rica has had a similar trajectory, with life expectancy trailing that of the US by nearly fifteen years in 1950 and matching or exceeding it since 1982.

Modern medicine can provide astonishingly effective prevention, care, and cure. But treatment programs often follow the "rule of halves"—they diagnose only half of patients, treat only half of those diagnosed, and provide effective treatment to only half of those treated.[35] This results in millions of preventable deaths. Thailand and Costa Rica improved health by investing in high-quality, accessible primary care for the most common health problems for virtually everyone. Despite its proven effectiveness, primary health care has little political power. Political and medical leaders give lip service to improving it, but less than 5 percent of Medicare expenditures in the US pay for primary care.[36] After twenty years of dedicated work, the average primary care practitioner in the US will earn less than half as much as a newly graduated surgeon.[37]

The weakness of primary health care in most countries, including the US, reflects the six drivers of the Cassandra curse. The *prevention paradox* undermines motivation to change: Small incremental improvements for large numbers of patients are imperceptible to individuals and not priority for most health care systems, even though they can result in larger improvements in community-wide health than dramatic, specialized care. *Powerful economic interests*, including hospitals and specialists, block our ability to see and then change health care finance to favor primary care. The *myth of unfettered free will* leads us to assume we're masters of our own health rather than recognize that without vaccines, treatments, screening, and follow-up, we may get sick and die. *Social norms* make effective solutions, such as more effective ways to organize and pay for health care, politically nonviable. *False alarms*, including news coverage of the latest scare or fad, desensitize us to the greatest real risks to our health and the need for accessible care. And *hyperbolic discounting*—shortchanging the future—leads people to underestimate and therefore be more likely to experience future suffering, and also leads health care systems to invest in short-term gains rather than longer-term improvements.[38] Although difficult, it's possible to overcome these barriers (see appendix 1 for a summary of barriers and means to overcome them).

Good primary health care implements the See part of the formula: It makes visible future devastating but preventable diseases. Many distressing conditions such as headaches, allergies, and rashes are far less likely to kill us than silent conditions such as high blood pressure, unhealthy cholesterol, or an insidiously growing cancer. What we want most from health care is often not what will help us most. Providers can see a ticking time bomb we may be unaware of—a small melanoma, an irregular heartbeat, high blood pressure. Primary health care providers also help patients see health crises that didn't happen. A wonderful pediatrician encouraged women to continue breastfeeding with a running patter during physical examinations of babies: "Healthy skin, because you're breastfeeding . . . healthy mucous membranes of the mouth and nose, because you're breastfeeding . . . clear lungs, because you're continuing to breastfeed." If the child was sick: "Just think how much sicker she'd be if you weren't breastfeeding!"

Cognitive behavioral therapy, a form of psychological counseling, helps patients recognize and overcome inaccurate perceptions and thought patterns that contribute to their problems.[39] Analogously, we can save lives if we recognize and counteract the drivers of the Cassandra curse. This allows us to more accurately see ourselves (including limitations on our free will and the social norms that shape our behavior), our world (influenced by economic interests, the prevention paradox, and false alarms), and the future (which we tend to undervalue because of hyperbolic discounting). Seeing and overcoming these forces can also help you protect your own health, as chapter 10 shows.

The final component of the See part of the formula, once we recognize invisible threats and overcome the barriers that prevent us from heeding warnings, is to use technical rigor to see the pathway to progress. "Follow the science" is a common plea, but it's misguided: Even where there's robust evidence, we must decide which solutions to choose and how to implement them. The next chapter shows how technical rigor enables us to uncover how disease spreads, interpret evidence correctly, prioritize, see the way forward, and implement effectively. This will complete the See portion of the formula, the essential first step to save the most lives.

3 THE PATHWAY TO PROGRESS

Science is the torch that illuminates the world.
—Louis Pasteur

"No Drama" President Obama was seething . . . at me, and the story was on the front page of the *New York Times*.[1] The world's first Ebola epidemic had been spreading in Guinea, Liberia, and Sierra Leone for months. The dramatic graph, described in chapter 1, had galvanized action. Teams from the CDC had surged into each country, tracking thousands of cases and tens of thousands of contacts from Ebola clusters, running laboratories, supporting emergency operations centers, and coordinating with governments, the World Health Organization, and others. In West Africa, the tide was beginning to turn, and in August 2014, in Lagos, Nigeria, the CDC had helped end a cluster of Ebola that could have become a continent-wide disaster. We thought we had averted the Cassandra prediction of future devastation. Then things went terribly wrong: We failed to use technical rigor in our analysis of how to prevent spread.

This failure with Ebola shows the importance of technical rigor: the ability to analyze complex health problems and understand both science and practical realities. The pathway to save the most lives might seem obvious—use the best available vaccines and medicines. But it's nowhere near that simple. Success requires nuanced understanding of evidence; practical tools to choose the right challenge, strategy, and tactics; and humility. This approach can transform facts and evidence into programs and progress.

THE PLURAL OF ANECDOTE IS NOT DATA

On September 15, 2014, Thomas Eric Duncan helped a sick, pregnant neighbor go to a hospital in Monrovia, Liberia. Five days later, he arrived in Texas to be with his partner and their children. Four days later—nine days after helping his pregnant neighbor—he went to the emergency department. The nurse documented that he had a high fever, and he told staff of his recent time in Liberia. Doctors missed the diagnosis of Ebola and sent Mr. Duncan home; when he returned three days later, he was deathly ill. During his care, two nurses, Nina Pham and Amber Vinson, became infected with Ebola.

Amber Vinson had visited her family in Ohio and then, while potentially infectious, with approval of a CDC staffer, taken a flight back to Texas along with people from dozens of other states. Our team needed to inform all these people that they might have been exposed to Ebola. It was the height of the 2014 midterm election season. There were calls for my resignation. The infections were a shock and a failure. A shock that the US is not immune to exotic health threats and a failure of CDC technical rigor to protect the nurses.

Confidence can inspire others to join efforts to save lives, but my biggest mistakes have come from overconfidence. Overconfidently, I had insisted that any US hospital could care for a patient with Ebola. I should have known better. After all, I had been infected—although not sickened—with the tuberculosis bacteria while caring for patients at a tuberculosis clinic in New York City, and those "pus bucket" hospitals had been the driving force behind the outbreak of multidrug-resistant tuberculosis in New York City in the 1990s.

How had CDC recommendations to protect health care workers from Ebola gone so wrong? Seeing the pathway to progress requires interpreting data correctly.

We thought we understood how to prevent the spread of Ebola in hospitals. We knew the virus spreads only by direct contact, not by the airborne route. CDC staff used only minimal precautions when they cared for Ebola patients in Africa in the 1970s, '80s, and '90s, and none became infected. Soap and water, bleach, and other disinfectants kill the virus easily.

We based our conclusions on cases of similar infections in the United States. In a remarkable coincidence, just a few days after Ebola emerged in West Africa, a man who had traveled from Liberia to Minnesota developed fever and confusion. Concerned, appropriately, about the possibility that he had Ebola, doctors sent specimens to the CDC lab in Atlanta; tests showed that he had Lassa fever. Lassa is in the same category as Ebola—a virus that can cause fatal bleeding and other complications.[2] The Minnesota patient was the fifth with Lassa fever treated in the United States in recent years. Not one of these patients spread Lassa to their family, their nurses, or their doctors, even though none had been diagnosed or isolated promptly. Health care workers hadn't used anything beyond routine gloves and handwashing. This gave us some reassurance that it wouldn't be too difficult to prevent the spread of Ebola in US hospitals. But an earlier, striking case figured much more prominently in our thinking.

On Christmas Day 2007, during a safari that included whitewater rafting and camping, a forty-four-year-old woman from Colorado hiked through dense vegetation and entered Python Cave in Queen Elizabeth Park, Uganda. She returned to Colorado on New Year's Day 2008. A week later, she became desperately ill. Her bone marrow, liver, and kidneys failed. Her blood didn't clot normally. The hospital sent her specimens to the CDC; all tests were negative.

Seven months later, while still recuperating, she read of a Dutch tourist who had visited the same cave in Uganda and later died from Marburg virus infection—an Ebola-like infection with a similarly high fatality rate and similar ways of spreading. She contacted the CDC; new blood tests confirmed Marburg infection. During her eleven-day hospital stay, dozens of health care workers had cared for her without any special isolation precautions. She had diarrhea, vomiting, and menstrual bleeding, had undergone multiple blood draws, and had intravenous lines placed and an operation to remove her gallbladder—and no one at the community hospital, which had used only standard gloves and handwashing, had been infected.[3] This—and the fact that no health care workers were infected by the Dutch patient with Marburg infection—gave us more confidence that routine precautions, if followed carefully, could protect health care workers from Ebola.

Stuart Nichol oversaw the CDC unit that tracked the source of the Colorado woman's Marburg infection. He's a kind, unflappable, wry, soft-spoken Englishman. He proudly showed me a photograph of their team examining bats captured in Python Cave following the call from Colorado. This investigation, together with a study at another cave months earlier, demonstrated that bats were the likely host reservoir of Marburg. Their team had gone into Python Cave to catch and study the bats. "Wasn't the team afraid?" I asked. "Well," Nichol said quietly, "they weren't afraid of Marburg because they were wearing those Tyvek suits and respirators. And they weren't afraid of the fifteen-foot python that lives there, feeding on the bats, because you could see it and avoid it. But they *were* scared of the cobras. There are lots of cobras on the floor of the cave, so they wore leather chaps underneath the space suits to protect them from the cobras." A newspaper clipping adorned the office door of the neighboring scientist who led the investigations: "MEN WANTED for hazardous journey, small wages, bitter cold, long months of complete darkness, constant danger, safe return doubtful, honor and recognition in case of success. Ernest Shackleton." The legendary explorer's ethos fit the team—except most prefer anonymity to recognition, and half were women. Nichol became the technical lead for the CDC response to the world's first Ebola epidemic.

We got our recommendations wrong in part because we didn't account for the vast difference between nursing care for Ebola in the United States and Africa. In Africa, staff of Ebola treatment units provided rudimentary care to patients who lay on plastic mattresses that were easy to disinfect. In Texas, the nurses washed, turned, and changed Mr. Duncan's bedclothes and sheets. On the day the two nurses likely became infected, Mr. Duncan had more than two and a half gallons of diarrhea, with trillions of virus particles, any one of which can cause infection. The nurses had never cared for a patient with Ebola. Unfamiliar with and understandably fearful of Ebola, they put on two or three layers of gloves, making it harder and more dangerous to remove the gloves without getting infected. The hospital hadn't given them appropriately fitted gowns, masks, and other protective equipment.

Also, we hadn't added a safety factor to correct for the fallibility of medical care. Doctors missed Mr. Duncan's Ebola diagnosis the first time he visited the hospital even though he had a high fever and told staff he had just come from Liberia. As a result, when he returned a few days later, he was much sicker and much more infectious.

We failed to protect health care workers because our recommendations relied on anecdotes and theories rather than evidence. Evidence would have warned us to be more careful: Infections that spread in US hospitals kill an estimated 70,000 people a year. But there's another, more intricate reason for our failure.

THE ART AND SCIENCE OF GETTING THE SCIENCE RIGHT

Technical rigor to see the path to progress requires a deep understanding of epidemiology. The two nurses might not have become infected if our recommendations had accounted for an important but little-known concept in disease transmission—*kappa*. *Kappa* shows that for some infectious diseases, a few people spread infection much more than others.

In contrast to the lesser-known *kappa*, the basic reproductive number, R_0, was used extensively—and excessively—to track COVID during the height of the pandemic. R_0 (pronounced *r-naught* or *r-zero*) can be useful—but also misused. The higher the R_0, the more rapid and extensive the spread. The movie *Contagion* shows a memorable explanation of R_0. Kate Winslet, playing a CDC epidemiologist, writes on a whiteboard to illustrate the concept to terrified local government leaders. She explains that if R_0 is below 1, each patient will infect less than one other patient and the infection will ultimately decrease or disappear. If R_0 is more than 1, the disease will spread, possibly to the entire world.

Karel Styblo, one of the most important scientists you've never heard of, had a profound understanding of tuberculosis, including how R_0 applies to its spread. In 1944, Nazi authorities imprisoned Styblo at the Mauthausen-Gusen concentration camp in Austria, where he contracted tuberculosis. Over the next forty years, as a doctor and epidemiologist, Styblo studied tuberculosis and learned to orchestrate all three parts of the formula. He saw invisible trends. He established the concept of a technical package based on scientific and practical rigor, as described later in this chapter. After a decade in Tanzania, he developed a powerful information system that can transform health care. He understood how the tuberculosis infection spreads among people. Even more importantly, he learned how to make a tuberculosis control program spread throughout a country, as described in chapter 6.

In January 1993, at the height of the outbreak of multidrug-resistant tuberculosis in New York City, Styblo explained to me over lunch in Chinatown how R_0 applies to tuberculosis. Drawing on a paper napkin (really), he explained that each tuberculosis patient, without treatment, infects on average fifteen people. Of those fifteen, 10 percent, or 1.5, develop tuberculosis. But of those, only half are highly infectious, so each case results, on average, in 0.75 cases likely to further spread the disease. "So you see," Styblo concluded, "the tuberculosis bacteria is doomed. It will disappear. But that will take two or three hundred years. Our job is to make it disappear faster."[4]

The R_0 of COVID in the initial wave was estimated to be 2–3, increasing to 10 during the Omicron wave; measles is believed to have the highest R_0 of any infection, 15–20.[5] Reality is more complex.[6] We don't know why, but some patients are much more infectious than others. To avoid stigmatizing people, we generally avoid the term "superspreaders," although in some situations it's accurate. (During one high-profile outbreak I explained the concept to Peter Madonia, Mayor Bloomberg's laconic, insightful chief of staff. He commented, "You mean, close-to-the-face talkers?" Maybe.) But R_0 is an average, and it doesn't capture a crucial aspect of the risk of spread: *kappa*—the wide variation in how infectious different patients are.[7]

In an ingenious experiment started in the 1950s and mentioned in chapter 1, scientists hermetically sealed the exhaust from hospital rooms of patients with tuberculosis. They vented all air through ducts and housed guinea pigs, which are highly susceptible to tuberculosis, in cages inside the ducts. They monitored patients and guinea pigs for years and made a startling discovery. A single patient hospitalized on the unit for just three days accounted for fifteen of twenty-nine guinea pig infections. This patient was more infectious than an average measles patient. Of sixty-one tuberculosis patients, all of whom in theory were highly infectious, fifty-three didn't cause a single guinea pig infection. A small proportion of patients accounted for the vast majority of infections.[8] *Kappa*—the dispersion factor—shows that a few patients are superspreaders and most won't ever spread their infection to anyone. Mr. Duncan, through no fault of his own, was highly infectious.[9]

Whether superspreading results from characteristics of the organism (a nasty strain), the patient (high microbial load), the environment (e.g., a poorly ventilated indoor space), behavior (e.g., singing), or a combination may differ by event and organism. If we had incorporated awareness of *kappa* into our recommendations for Ebola precautions in US hospitals, we would have protected workers not from the average patient but from the most infectious patient—someone like Mr. Duncan.[10]

Kappa and other rigorous analytic tools can help identify the path to disease control—the See part of the formula. But sometimes we have to figure out how to stop a disease that arises mysteriously. A year before I was born, my parents lost their healthy three-month-old son—their third child—to "crib death," sudden infant death syndrome (SIDS). Without a remarkable study, you or your children might have shared my late brother's fate.

EVIDENCE AND PROOF

Ed Mitchell was born in Iran and went to elementary school in South Yemen. His parents were British; his father, a mechanical engineer, fixed oil refinery pumps. Becoming a doctor in London, Mitchell got fed up with the hierarchical nature of British medicine and society and moved to New Zealand. Just before he arrived, the health department noticed a high death rate among infants in the community. Mitchell's department at the University of Auckland School of Medicine was under pressure to find the cause and fix it. As the most junior member of the team, Mitchell was assigned the task of reviewing the out-of-hospital deaths. Studying the children who had died in the community "was a complete eye-opener." Hospital review committees assessed deaths from leukemia, pneumonia, and other conditions, but these deaths were, fortunately, rare. What he found in the community stunned Mitchell—many infants died suddenly and unexpectedly. These deaths had been invisible to him and to the other doctors, who provided care only for infants at the hospital. "We kept hearing the same story. It was heartbreaking. Babies who went to sleep perfectly healthy dying from no apparent cause." These deaths were mysterious tragedies.

For years, Dr. Shirley Tonkin, an Auckland health department doctor, visited families whose infants had died at home. She noticed that many apparently healthy babies had been placed to sleep on their stomach, an observation Dr. Susan Beal had also made. At Tonkin's insistence, Mitchell included sleep position in the review of infant deaths.

This review confirmed that many infants who died suddenly had been placed on their stomach to sleep. Although intriguing, this didn't prove anything. Maybe all babies were put to sleep this way. To discover whether sleep position was the cause of the deaths, it was necessary to have a comparison group—infants who didn't die. Mitchell's group began a three-year case-control study to explore this and other possibilities.[11]

On sabbatical in London shortly after the first year of the study, Mitchell tried to make sense of the data. "As a pediatrician, I couldn't believe something as simple as placing babies prone could increase the risk of sudden death substantially. Basically thought it was rubbish."[12] He consulted a prominent statistician, who jotted calculations on the back of an envelope: Most cases of SIDS were attributable to putting babies on their stomach to sleep.[13] This was stunning: It's rare for a simple risk to account for more than half of deaths from any cause. Although the evidence wasn't definitive, it was strong enough for the New Zealand government to educate parents to put infants on their back to sleep. SIDS deaths then declined spectacularly, proving that back-sleeping prevents SIDS.[14] We still don't know why prone-sleeping increases SIDS risk. A randomized controlled trial (RCT) would have taken years and been unlikely to result in a definitive outcome. SIDS is rare, adherence by parents to a randomized recommendation of back-sleeping would have been impractical, and it would be unethical to randomize babies to prone-sleeping when this could increase the risk of SIDS.

"Evidence-based programs"—in plain English, programs proven to work by RCTs or other methods—are important. But public health often advances because of something very different: program-based evidence. A promising program, such as New Zealand's back-to-sleep campaign, gets implemented, rigorously evaluated, and proves what works. Both practice-based evidence and evidence-based practice are examples of the technical rigor needed to see the pathway to progress.

To compare two medications, a placebo-controlled, double- (or triple-) blinded RCT is often ideal. In such a study, patients are randomly allocated to different groups and receive different treatment. Neither the patient nor the doctor (nor, in the case of triple-blinding, the statistician analyzing the results) knows which patients received which treatment. Many researchers have the misconception that RCTs, which seem perfect, are the best form of evidence. They aren't.[15] RCTs are unlikely to measure outcomes that require years of follow-up—for example, how long vaccines protect or the decades-long impact of treatment. The trials usually take years to complete and are expensive. For rare diseases, there aren't enough patients to randomly assign a sufficient number to different treatment groups, so RCTs can't be done. And RCTs can be wrong.

A nasal spray influenza vaccine was licensed in 2003; by 2014 several RCTs had shown it to be superior to other influenza vaccines for healthy children two to eight years old. The following year, observational studies showed the vaccine to be no better than other vaccines. Subsequently, the vaccine was found to have no effectiveness at all against the most common strain of influenza and was not recommended until the manufacturer reformulated it.[16] Whether changes in the vaccine, the virus, or immunity levels caused this reversal isn't clear, but it is clear that the RCT was less accurate than observational studies. (Formally, this is an example of "internal validity"—the RCT was correct for the population in which it was studied but had low "external validity," with findings not relevant for people exposed to influenza after the trial was over.) RCTs are just one form of evidence.

Much of clinical medicine hasn't been studied by RCTs. This is the dark matter of clinical medicine: Like dark matter in the universe, there's much more of it than the few bright spots. For many public health questions, an RCT is neither practical nor the most reliable source of knowledge. For example, taxing tobacco reduces smoking, but it would be difficult or impossible to design an RCT to prove this. There's no single, best approach to study health interventions; clinicians and public health specialists must almost always make decisions based on careful analysis and interpretation of imperfect data.[17]

Even well-conducted studies may become irrelevant if the population, pathogen, or context changes. Dr. George Comstock was one of the top epidemiologists of the twentieth century, superbly talented and methodical and also humble, soft-spoken, and gentle. He started his career in Alaska demonstrating rapid control of tuberculosis. Comstock's classic studies showed that one in ten people infected with the tuberculosis bacteria developed active disease, with about half developing tuberculosis in the two years after infection.[18] Decades later, he wrote an article calling for studies on this very question.[19] I puzzled about why he suggested that others repeat his studies; he couldn't have forgotten the results of his own studies. Did he know of some error in his methods? I was too embarrassed to ask him until many years later. His response: "That was then, this is now. The bacteria might have changed. The nutritional status of infected people might have changed. The inoculum [the number of bacteria that infect a person] might have changed. We won't know unless we study it." It's not enough to understand the findings of a study; scientists like Comstock see more deeply into methods and contexts and understand the need to interpret findings with caution.

Some advocates of evidence-based medicine don't agree that data analysis is an art and a science, informed by rigorous analysis of all relevant data, including the strengths and limitations of each individual study. When I made this point publicly, a prominent proponent of the evidence-based medicine line of reasoning commented, "Baloney, absolutely baloney."[20]

Getting the right answer requires going beyond RCTs and beyond structured reviews; it requires assessment of each piece of evidence's strengths, weaknesses, and relevance. An RCT might not apply to a current situation. Meta-analyses and systematic reviews can err without deep knowledge of the quality and applicability of individual studies. Real rigor requires blending methodological precision with the insights of a specialist—someone like George Comstock—to understand both the value and the limitations of evidence.[21]

Another common and deadly failure of technical rigor occurs in studies that suggest that small amounts of a substance are good, but too much is bad.

These studies describe a J-shaped relationship between exposure and death, with the best outcomes at the bottom of the J, with a little exposure, higher death rates among people with no exposure, and rates increasing starting above the sweet spot of a little exposure. This was claimed for alcohol—the assertion that people who drink a little live longer. There's just one problem with studies that find a J-shaped relationship between exposures and health outcomes: They're usually wrong. This error is caused by *confounding*: A factor causes both the lowest level of consumption and negative health outcomes. People who don't drink include those ill from prior heavy drinking and people too ill to drink. This group has a higher death rate than light drinkers not because alcohol is healthy but because their underlying health is worse. Poor health is the confounder—causing both higher mortality and avoidance of alcohol.

In some studies, lower blood pressure is associated with higher mortality; when analyzed accurately, these studies show that blood pressure declines as overall health declines. This decline is the confounding factor that causes both lower blood pressure and higher risk of death.[22] The spurious association between low consumption and a bad outcome can also result from inaccurate measurement at low levels. In the case of sodium consumption, erroneous calculations suggested a J-shaped relationship. Accurate measurement shows that the relationship is linear—the lower the sodium, the better the health outcomes.[23]

There are a few true J-shaped associations. Too little of vitamins A and D causes vision, skin, and bone problems. Too much causes broken bones, seizures, and other neurological problems. It's almost impossible to get too much of these two vitamins from food; nearly all toxicity results from taking too many vitamin supplements. (One exception: Inuit populations that consume blubber rich in vitamins A and D.[24])

Disagreements over how to interpret evidence also reflect the different worldviews of clinical medicine and public health. Both consider risks and benefits, but doctors assess potential outcomes for individual patients; public health specialists consider consequences for entire communities. Doctors see normal human physiology as the baseline and require strong proof to change something that has worked well for millennia. Public health specialists see the current situation as shaped by past choices—many harmful—by companies, governments, and others, and act when a new policy can improve health.

Figuring out what works to solve a health problem is important, but to save the most lives, deciding which problems to solve—the first of three tools of technical rigor—is also essential.

BURDEN × AMENABILITY: A TOOL FOR PRIORITIZATION

Deciding on the health problems to address may seem easy, but it's not. Many well-meaning programs fail to prevent much illness, suffering, or death. A rigorous tool shows the way forward: The burden of a disease multiplied by its amenability to prevention or control, Burden × Amenability. Burden—how many people suffer from a condition—is important, but saving the most lives requires tackling problems that have a large burden and can be stopped through focused action.

Consider breast cancer, smoking, and hypertension. Each has a high global burden, killing 700,000, 8 million, and 11 million people a year, respectively. More than 2 million women are diagnosed with breast cancer every year.[25] Although mammograms can detect cancer early and improve survival,[26] the unfortunate reality is that mammography is a weak tool, even with innovations of digital imaging and artificial intelligence. Even with regular mammography and complete follow-up, most breast cancers won't be prevented, and many women will undergo stressful biopsies and other potentially harmful procedures because of falsely positive images.[27] With clinical support—counseling and medication—smokers are twice as likely to quit. But even with the best medication and counseling, most smokers who try to quit fail. In contrast, hypertension treatment greatly reduces the risk of stroke, heart attack, heart failure, kidney failure, and dementia.

Of course clinical systems should provide high-quality mammography and follow-up. And of course doctors should counsel smokers to quit and prescribe medications to help. But using the Burden × Amenability formula, although the burden of all three conditions—breast cancer, smoking, and hypertension—is high, the number of lives that can be saved by medical treatment is by far highest for hypertension. Improving blood pressure control will save many more lives than improving mammography or smoking-cessation counseling.[28] We can save the most lives if we fund research to improve prevention and cure of breast cancer, tax tobacco, and improve treatment of hypertension.

Many health planners and advocates object to focusing on a limited set of services. It's unethical, they say, to focus on only some of the things that save lives. The phrase "progressive universalism" in health care coverage finesses this issue: steadily increasing coverage, starting with the highest-impact services for those most in need and expanding to more people and more conditions as human and financial resources allow.[29] It's certainly true that every provider should try to provide optimal care for every patient. But as Hans Rosling wrote: "So long as resources are not infinite—and they never are infinite—it is the most compassionate thing to do to use your brain and work out how to do the most good with what you have."[30] This is not a dry, theoretical debate. Those trying to "do everything" run well-meaning but poorly thought-out programs that have limited impact. In contrast, a strategic approach identifies the most important conditions and can substantially reduce suffering, disability, and death.

THE HEALTH IMPACT PYRAMID: A TOOL TO GUIDE STRATEGY

Technical rigor reveals how to interpret evidence accurately, and the Burden × Amenability calculation shows how to choose programs that can save the most lives. But that's not enough. The health impact pyramid (figure 3.1)[31] is a tool to identify the most effective approach; the largest health benefit comes from actions at the lowest level where progress is feasible.

The bottom tier, including improvements in education and the economy, and the second-lowest tier, including clean air and clean water, require law and regulation; change may be slow and, at times, politically impossible.[32] Care at the middle level necessitates reaching people individually with long-lasting interventions, but the impact can be large: Global

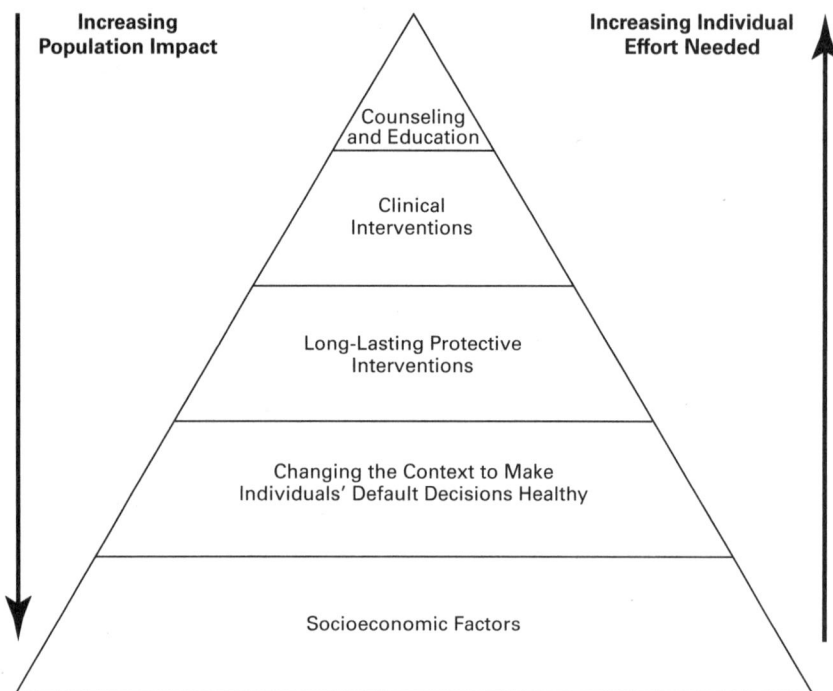

Increasing Population Impact

Increasing Individual Effort Needed

Counseling and Education

Clinical Interventions

Long-Lasting Protective Interventions

Changing the Context to Make Individuals' Default Decisions Healthy

Socioeconomic Factors

Figure 3.1

The health impact pyramid. Actions lower on the pyramid require more collective effort and less individual effort, have a greater impact, and are generally harder to get enacted. Reproduced with permission from Thomas R. Frieden, "A Framework for Public Health Action: The Health Impact Pyramid," *American Journal of Public Health* 100, no. 4 (February 19, 2010): 590–595.

immunization programs prevent millions of childhood deaths each year.[33] The second-highest level of the pyramid represents ongoing clinical interventions. Impact is limited by lack of access, low patient adherence, imperfect treatment effectiveness, and poorly performing health care systems. The pyramid's smallest, top tier represents health education. Public health is sometimes seen as the annoying nag telling people to eat their vegetables, sit up straight, do calisthenics. In New York City coffee shops, a "double no-fun" is a decaffeinated coffee with a sugar substitute. Sadly, many people consider public health a double no-fun. But promoting changes in individual behaviors is not the core of public health—it's a symptom of public health failure. It's not necessary to tell people in countries with safe water to boil and filter it to prevent intestinal infections. When public health succeeds, societal changes make the individuals' default choices healthy.

Hypertension illustrates how to see invisible threats, use the Burden × Amenability calculation, and apply the impact pyramid. Hypertension is the most lethal, neglected, and pervasive pandemic of our time; deaths are largely invisible precisely because they are so common. Many people assume, incorrectly, that increased blood pressure and the resulting premature deaths are a normal part of aging—the illusion of inevitability. With every heartbeat, every second of every day, high blood pressure pounds like a battering ram on artery walls in the heart, brain, kidneys, and throughout the body. High blood pressure causes more than one out of every six deaths. Because hypertension is easily treatable, it scores highly on the Burden × Amenability calculation.

Improved socioeconomic status, the lowest level of the pyramid, might decrease the proportion of people who have hypertension, although change is likely to be slow and not easy to achieve.[34] Changing the default choice, the second-lowest level of the pyramid—for example, through promotion of potassium-enriched low-sodium salt—can reduce blood pressure and prevent heart attacks and strokes.[35] Countries can regulate to reduce sodium consumption: stop-sign-like front-of-pack warnings; mandatory limits on unhealthy salt levels; bans on marketing and promotion; and taxes on unhealthy foods. Implementing these effective policies requires overcoming opposition from powerful food manufacturing companies. Progress will be faster if healthy food, such as vegetables, fruit, and potassium-enriched salt, is more affordable and available.[36]

The middle level of the pyramid—one-time or long-lasting interventions—is less relevant to hypertension. Intriguing but inconclusive data suggest that providing healthier sodium levels to infants may result in healthier choices many years later.[37] A vaccine to prevent or treat high blood pressure isn't yet available. Newer interventions that could make this tier relevant are being studied: surgery to reduce blood pressure by cutting nerves going to the kidneys, and injections that reduce blood pressure for up to six months.[38] The top of the pyramid—counseling individuals—has almost no impact reducing blood pressure.[39] Encouraging people to eat less salt—without changing the food environment—generally doesn't work.[40] Despite challenges, treatment has great potential to save lives from hypertension.

For every twenty-point increase in blood pressure starting at 115/75, the risk of death from a heart attack or stroke doubles.[41] (The first number is the systolic pressure—the highest pressure in the arteries when the heart squeezes blood out—and the second is the diastolic, the lowest pressure when the heart ventricles relax.) Although higher blood pressure starting at a systolic measurement of 115 correlates with higher mortality, until recently it hadn't been proven that reducing blood pressure to this level with medications benefits patients. A meticulous RCT has now demonstrated that treatment with a systolic pressure target of 120 substantially reduces heart attacks, strokes, and deaths compared to a target of 140.[42] Better treatment of hypertension can save more than a million lives a year.

A disease detective's report from 1848 illustrates how the pyramid works. The Prussian government sent Rudolph Virchow, a famous pathologist, to investigate a massive typhus epidemic. He failed to identify the organism—bacteriology was rudimentary back then—but did identify the cause and cure of the health crisis. He advised land reform, crop rotation, education, workers' rights, and democracy.[43]

In a parable told to public health students, a river runs through a village, and suddenly a child thrashes by, nearly drowning, swept down the river. Townspeople rush to rescue the child. Then another child comes struggling down, and another, and another. The rescuers can hardly keep up, and suddenly one man turns around and runs away from the river. "Where are you going?" the shocked townspeople ask. "Upstream to find out how they're falling in and stop them." That's public health.

TECHNICAL PACKAGES: A TOOL TO FOCUS EFFORT

Rigorous analysis, systematic priority-setting, and choosing the right level of intervention are just the start. Consider tuberculosis. It's high burden—more than a million deaths every year. It has been curable since the 1950s. The impact pyramid identifies treatment as the most efficient way to save lives at present. But for nearly half a century after doctors discovered the cure, tuberculosis deaths continued to increase, until 1993—a turning point.

In 1993, tuberculosis experts at the World Health Organization (WHO) released a structured, simple *technical package*: a limited number of specific, synergistic interventions. Stopping tuberculosis had been complicated and overwhelming. As an infectious disease specialist treating tuberculosis patients and overseeing the New York City control program, I debated issues such as which medicines to prescribe, which masks health care workers should use, and which laboratory tests to order. These controversies were intellectually interesting, but Dr. Karel Styblo, with his decades of experience and clear vision of the way forward, taught us that the answers made little difference. Dozens of activities could be the focus of efforts to stop tuberculosis, but the pathway to progress was a few interventions—the technical package. Any part of the package would be insufficient, and diluting the package with additional, lower-priority activities would make progress slower and less likely. A technical package based on the best science and the best practical experience avoids vague commitments to "action" that result in a scattershot approach that tries to do everything for everyone but accomplishes little for anyone.[44]

Styblo's technical package for tuberculosis control, known as DOTS, consists of five components: political commitment, good quality diagnosis, reliable drug supply, good quality treatment, and a simple but extraordinarily powerful information system.[45] DOTS focuses the attention of health care workers, supervisors, and program managers on the essentials: accurate diagnosis, complete treatment, and monitoring the outcome of every patient's treatment. Tuberculosis treatment programs in more than one hundred countries use nearly identical records. This makes training, diagnosis, medication procurement, treatment, monitoring, comparison among countries, and effective supervision much easier. WHO focused on implementing a minimal number of effective policies in the countries with the most tuberculosis. It became possible for WHO, country programs, and partners to train thousands of leaders and hundreds of thousands of health care workers, cure tens of millions of patients, and begin to reverse the global tuberculosis epidemic. The result: After WHO launched the DOTS program in 1993, the death rate from tuberculosis decreased by 60 percent, saving more than thirty million lives in the following 30 years.[46]

A philanthropic initiative begun by Mike Bloomberg while he was New York City Mayor shows the power of a technical package to reduce tobacco use. Tobacco control activists seemed to spend most of their time fighting about a few controversial issues rather than implementing what everyone agreed on. Bloomberg supported WHO to launch a technical package— MPOWER—that consists of six measures: monitoring tobacco use; protecting people from tobacco smoke with smoke-free laws; offering help to quit; warning about the dangers of tobacco; enforcing bans on advertising, promotion, and sponsorship; and, most importantly, raising prices, primarily through taxation. Partnering with WHO, activists, and country leadership, the effort has supported programs that will prevent more than 35 million deaths.[47]

Technical packages can focus action on manageable goals. Trans fat, previously the main ingredient in margarine, was introduced into the food supply in the latter half of the twentieth century. It prolongs the shelf life of food and makes pie crusts crispy. Unfortunately, it's solid not only in pie crusts but also in coronary arteries, and was responsible for up to 500,000 deaths every year. REPLACE, the technical package WHO and Resolve to Save Lives created to eliminate trans fat, now covers most of the world's population and will prevent more than 10 million deaths from heart disease in the next twenty-five years.[48] Instead of vague advice to "eat healthy" or complex advice on what to eat and what not to eat, the simple approach of using a focused technical package to eliminate an artificial, toxic compound has enabled rapid global progress.

A technical package can help control the world's leading cause of death, hypertension. The Burden × Amenability calculation summarized above identifies hypertension as an important area. The health impact pyramid shows that medical treatment can save millions of lives now. Resolve to Save Lives worked with WHO and others to establish HEARTS, a technical package that includes protocol-driven treatment, team-based and patient-centered care, and a Styblo-inspired information system.

It's not easy to get a technical package accepted and implemented. Some doctors criticize the protocols HEARTS recommends as "cookbook medicine." A protocol is a set of specific drugs and doses with a step-by-step schedule to start, increase, and add medications. Rigorous studies in the 1970s demonstrated that nurses following protocols controlled blood pressure more effectively than cardiologists who used their clinical judgment.[49] The findings didn't surprise my father, who had observed, "When you see how some doctors practice medicine, you realize how resilient the human body is." In the US and globally, protocols have saved millions of lives from HIV, tuberculosis, childhood diseases, and more. Artificial intelligence has the potential to further increase health benefits by optimizing protocols and increasing the likelihood that providers select the right protocol for the right patient.

Team-based and patient-centered care—when doctors work with nurses, pharmacists, and others to ensure convenient, effective treatment—is essential. This is particularly important for conditions such as hypertension that have no symptoms and require long-term treatment; at least a third of patients don't take medications as prescribed.[50] Information systems that use the Styblo logic can drive progress. Doctors in many health care systems believe their patients are treated effectively, but community surveys reveal low control rates. The difference occurs because many high-risk patients aren't in care, clinical quality indicators exclude too many patients, and information systems are inaccurate. In the United Kingdom, the clinical indicator reported more than 80 percent blood pressure control, but community-wide surveys showed that less than 40 percent of people with hypertension had it under control.[51] Every effective technical package includes accurate and timely monitoring of program performance and impact, the part of public health's surveillance superpower that makes progress or failure visible.

HUMILITY

Technical rigor doesn't lead to certainty—it engenders humility. In February of 2020, it became horrifyingly clear that COVID would spread widely.

An outbreak on the Diamond Princess cruise ship in late January 2020 and reports of many health care workers and patients contracting the virus in hospitals in China showed that the virus was highly infectious.[52] The finding that many people with the infection didn't have symptoms was particularly ominous—containing the virus would be impossible.[53] In a press briefing on February 5, 2020, Dr. Nancy Messonnier of the CDC had exactly the right message and wording to frame the unavoidable uncertainties:

> Despite the years of planning, we need to remain humble and understand that we may not have planned for everything. We expect to see additional cases of novel coronavirus in the United States among returning travelers as well as their close contacts.[54]

No matter how rigorous public health analysis is, as we learn more, we may change our conclusions. Certainty is the Achilles' heel of science.[55] When asked later during the same press conference whether she was confident about the global situation, she answered in words that could hardly be improved, even many years later, for their frank admission of incomplete knowledge, recognition of the potential for damage, call to action, and message of hope:

> I think that this comes down to the need to be humble. . . . I don't think that we've seen that right now there is any sign that this has stopped. I think that it is premature to comment on whether it has slowed down. But we do believe that we have a window of opportunity now to prepare the United States in case that there is a broader spread of this outside China as well as a broader spread in the United States. And so as I said before, we're preparing as if this is a pandemic. That is just good common-sense public health. But of course I'm hoping that it is not.[56]

On February 10, 2020, President Donald Trump said, "We're in great shape," and "It's going to be fine."[57] Nothing could have been further from the truth—or from Dr. Messonnier's appropriate message of humility.

Using technical rigor, science searches for better answers, not immutable truths. Technical rigor requires a deep understanding of the topic, its relation to other areas of health and society, and the realities of implementation. Sometimes technical rigor means understanding what's really happening between patients and health care workers—how nurses put on and take off their gloves, whether patients are taking medicines as prescribed, or how health care workers and the public use masks. It requires humility to be open to new evidence and to change policies when this evidence changes our understanding. On the first day of medical school, the dean told our class that half of all they taught us was wrong, but they didn't know which half so would test us on all. Since then, for example, use of one type of medication—beta blockers—in patients with a weakened heart muscle has been transformed from something considered malpractice to give to something now considered malpractice *not* to give.[58]

Technical rigor requires deep analysis of scientific evidence integrated with a nuanced understanding of practical realities. With that foundation, the Burden × Amenability calculation helps identify high-impact initiatives. The health impact pyramid reveals the most effective strategy. Technical packages focus implementation on what works. Applying these tools requires scientific precision, pragmatism, and humility.

But even with technical rigor, there's a critical gap between knowing what to do and getting it done: Believing that change is possible. The See part of the formula reveals trends in microbes, communities, toxic exposures, and program progress (chapter 1), recognizes forces that make us ignore warnings (chapter 2), and enables us to see the pathway to progress by showing how to understand disease spread, interpret evidence, prioritize, and find solutions that save lives (the current chapter). Technical rigor is also vital for personal health—to reveal the pathway to a long, healthy life, as chapter 10 shows. But disease and suffering often seem inescapable. Unless we break that illusion of inevitability, even the best-designed programs will fail.

For decades, governments have starved public health of funding. In 2025, the US spent $15,000 per person on health care but fifty times less—around $300 per person—on public health. State and local public health departments have lost funding, staff, and legal authorities. The White House, Department of Health and Human Services, and Congress all pillaged the Prevention and Public Health Fund, intended to increase resources for the CDC, to fund other programs.[59] And that was *before* the COVID pandemic resulted in a devastating decrease in trust of and support for public health, and before the second Trump administration cut US and global public health programs and institutions.

Although public health has done great things in the past, there may be a lurking suspicion that the world has become too complex, bureaucratic, conflicted, or inefficient to fight and win great battles. Chapter 4 shows how to implement the Believe part of the formula, the next essential step to save the most lives.

PART II BELIEVE

PART II BELIEVE

4 BELIEVE IN A HEALTHY FUTURE

The future belongs to those who believe in the beauty of their dreams.
—attributed to Eleanor Roosevelt

Tiny sores on Egyptian mummies are the first evidence of smallpox, a disease that caused high fevers, lesions that developed into pus, and sores that bled at the slightest touch, rotting the body and emanating the stench of death.[1] Along with measles and other infections, smallpox decimated Indigenous people in North America, spread in part by contaminated blankets given by settlers.[2] Although George Washington's troops outnumbered the British during the Battle of Quebec at the end of 1775, a smallpox outbreak so debilitated American forces that they lost. In 1777, at the urging of Benjamin Franklin and others, Washington ordered smallpox variolation (an earlier, less safe form of inoculation) of all troops.[3] If Washington hadn't ordered variolation when he did, America might have lost the Revolutionary War. If he had ordered it two years earlier, Canada might have become part of the United States.

Dr. Bill Foege helped lead smallpox eradication efforts in Nigeria and India. Facing a shortage of vaccine in Nigeria, Foege imagined what he would do if he were a smallpox virus: He'd try to infect people closest to him, then break through to other areas. Using this insight, he created a new approach called surveillance and containment. The prior strategy—mass vaccination—was neither necessary nor efficient. With the new strategy, teams identified and stopped previously invisible chains of transmission.

They found all smallpox cases—possible because of the obvious skin lesions—then isolated infected people, quarantined and vaccinated their closest contacts, and vaccinated people in surrounding communities.[4] Through these efforts, Foege revolutionized the world's approach to combating smallpox.

In his wonderful book, *House on Fire*, Foege describes how teams innovated with everything from ring vaccination and needles to meetings, progress reports, and educational messages.[5] He became a highly successful director of the CDC, was founding director of the Carter Center, which has prevented suffering of tens of millions of people, and helped start the Bill and Melinda Gates Foundation, catalyzing creation of a vaccine alliance that has saved more than 15 million lives. The witty, fast-thinking, eloquent, six-feet-seven-inch man who survived three usually fatal health conditions is in a league of his own.

Foege had applied the See part of the formula. Improved surveillance—the public health superpower—revealed thousands of smallpox outbreaks and showed where the disease was spreading. He established the technical package: isolation of patients with smallpox, ring vaccination of people who might have been in contact with cases, and active search for new smallpox cases. Smallpox topped the Burden × Amenability formula: It killed millions of people annually and public health action could drive those deaths to zero. A vaccine—the middle layer of the impact pyramid—was available and inexpensive. But doctors and communities around the world saw smallpox as inevitable. It would have been impossible to mobilize the massive effort and resources needed to eradicate smallpox unless he convinced others that success was possible. At its peak, the effort relied on more than 200,000 health care workers in more than seventy countries to find and vaccinate tens of millions of potential contacts. Asked for his job description, Foege responded: "Resident con man. My job is to keep people believing—'We can do this!'"

Foege's role as "resident con man" highlighted a central challenge: How can we implement the Believe part of the formula and overcome the presumption that disease is inevitable? First, show that progress has happened before.

CELEBRATE PAST PROGRESS

Before its eradication in 1979, smallpox killed more than half a billion people. It's unlikely that even one of the 8 billion people in the world today woke up this morning and thought, "Thank goodness I didn't die from smallpox yesterday." The smallpox program made the disease—widely feared for centuries and resulting in deep, conspicuous pockmarks on the face of survivors—invisible. Starting from a baseline of approximately 10 million cases a year with outbreaks in thirty-one countries in 1967, the last natural smallpox case occurred just a decade later. Smallpox eradication is one of the greatest achievements of public health—and of humanity. It has saved millions of lives and billions of dollars.[6]

A history of the New York City Health Department noted, in wise words I've kept on my desk for decades:

> Encountering apathy, ignorance, and avarice is the lot of all conscientious health officers. As preventive measures in the health area are more successful, the public is less inclined to support the programs which ensure this success.[7]

The public health curse is even more severe than Cassandra's—people ignore not only warnings of future devastation but also the lives saved from past tragedies prevented. Because of hyperbolic discounting, we shortchange not only the future but also the past. In 1923, C.-E. A. Winslow, a cofounder of the American Public Health Association, observed—in imagined situations that express the invisibility of progress—the "silent victories" of public health:

> If we had but the gift of second sight to transmute abstract figures into flesh and blood, so that as we walk along the street we could say "That man would be dead of typhoid fever," "That woman would have succumbed to tuberculosis," "That rosy infant would be in its coffin,"—then only should we have a faint conception of the meaning of the silent victories of public health.[8]

We tend to romanticize the past.[9] For much of human history, infectious diseases sickened, disabled, or killed people. Most children who survived had stunted physical and cognitive growth. Public health progress makes today's world look very different.

A periodic report published by Resolve to Save Lives titled *Epidemics That Didn't Happen* highlights work of health workers who stop outbreaks when and where they emerge. In the United States, we take for granted—although it's not always the case—that our water won't contain cholera bacteria, lead, or other harmful microbes or toxins. Without the substantial investments we've made in safe water for more than a century, debilitating and deadly waterborne outbreaks would be common, as they remain in far too many parts of the world today. Every time doctors and public health programs treat a patient for tuberculosis, gonorrhea, HIV, hepatitis, strep throat, and other infections they may be preventing an outbreak.

The first step to shatter the illusion of inevitability is to show that the world has already made lots of progress. Seeing past progress is an essential component of the Believe part of the formula. Public health staff are often reluctant to discuss progress in the face of the need for continued or intensified efforts. Hans Rosling revealed this tendency in his book *Factfulness*. Heroically, Rosling wrote the book in the last year of his life after being diagnosed with incurable pancreatic cancer. He knew his time was short and tried to convey the most important lessons learned from his lifetime of work in public health. He noted that it's hard to hold two contradictory ideas in our mind—that a condition is much better than before but still bad: "Things can be both bad and better. . . . Better, and bad, at the same time."[10]

Celebrating past progress doesn't have to mean declaring victory. Iodized salt protects 20 million children a year from developmental disability, but millions remain at risk for brain damage from maternal iodine deficiency.[11] Lead contamination has decreased in the US and leaded gasoline is a risk of the past, but lead continues to poison millions of people. Folate fortification of wheat and other foods has prevented hundreds of thousands of babies from having a severe congenital brain anomaly, but insufficient maternal folate continues to cause preventable severe problems for tens of thousands of children every year. Deficiencies of vitamins B3 and D previously caused common problems with skin and bones that are now essentially gone from the US but persist in many parts of the world. Properly framed, past progress doesn't lead to complacency but fuels momentum, urgency, and belief in the possibility of progress.

Recognizing progress is also important to prevent recurrence of past disasters. Progress against measles is invisible in the United States because the disease is largely gone. Before vaccination, in many years, measles infected millions of children in the US, left thousands blind, deaf, or disabled, and killed hundreds. Vaccination reduced cases and, as part of rapid public health action to detect and respond to outbreaks, eliminated spread within the US by the year 2000.[12] Recent outbreaks in the US result in avoidable illness and death and reflect both misinformation about vaccines and the difficulty of helping people see threats that were once vivid but now seem remote. Global vaccination has prevented millions of deaths, but low vaccination coverage results in measles killing more than 100,000 children around the world each year and stunting the development of millions more.[13] Seeing past progress stopping measles can help prevent a resurgence.

An illusion of inevitability distorts our understanding of illness and death; the Believe part of the formula shatters that illusion. Past victories—over infectious diseases, toxins, injuries, and disability—demonstrate that public health can save millions of lives. There's a systematic way to further strengthen belief in the potential for progress.

PHASE OUT THE FALSE SENSE OF INEVITABILITY

Celebrating past progress can seem naïve in the face of current challenges. New York City's tuberculosis outbreak had been overwhelming with 3,000 cases a year. In 1996, when I moved to India, the country had an estimated 3 million cases a year. Stopping an epidemic 1,000 times larger than New York City's was inconceivable.

There's nothing scarier than knowing that your actions might help determine whether millions of people live or die. India had every reason to succeed: Strategic leadership, a large World Bank loan, and support from the WHO unit that had many of the world's best tuberculosis experts. But progress was glacial, despite India's expertise; India had conducted many foundational investigations on tuberculosis. Decades earlier, a director general of WHO observed, "The whole world benefits from the fruits of Indian tuberculosis research. The whole world, except India." Leaving the antiquated health ministry building at ten most nights, I would curse myself: "Today tuberculosis killed 1,000 people in India, and what the f--- did I do about it?" I felt frustrated and overwhelmed.

Vaishali, Bihar, is a quick flight then drive from Delhi, India's capital. In the mid-1990s, Bihar was the Wild West of India, with violence, few functioning government institutions, and some of the worst health outcomes and health system performance in the country. Although Vaishali is renowned for delicious lychee fruit and as the place the Buddha is said to have found enlightenment, it seemed an inauspicious place for a new tuberculosis control program. The district tuberculosis officer, Dr. Gautam Vir, selected government staff known as multipurpose workers for the critical role of supporting tuberculosis patients. This wasn't a promising choice: These staff were disaffected and epitomized the line heard from government staff in many countries: "You pretend to pay us and we pretend to work."

Dr. Vir is smart, thoughtful, and sincere. Having survived polio as a child, he dragged one leg along with the help of a gnarled wooden stick. He provided the motivation—persuading, cajoling, and ordering workers to help. At first, they refused, but they gradually realized that the tuberculosis program Styblo had designed gave them status: For the first time, they had medicines that could cure patients.

One year after the Vaishali program started, the multipurpose workers, who hadn't been paid in months, went on strike. They refused to do any of their assigned tasks. Any, that is, except treat patients with tuberculosis. There was a reason they were willing to continue to provide medications. In Bihar, tuberculosis was common but almost no treatment had been available. Perhaps the most disturbing place I saw among the hundreds of health care facilities I assessed in India was Bihar's state tuberculosis center. The roof was caved in, the walls broken, and the pharmacy nearly empty. Nevertheless, starting at five in the morning, patients from all over the large state lined up, desperate for care. Worse, the center had only one medication to treat tuberculosis patients, not the three or four needed. This guaranteed that many patients would develop drug-resistant tuberculosis and few would be cured. The average weight of an adult tuberculosis patient at diagnosis was a skeletal ninety-two pounds—patients were dying of tuberculosis as they had a century earlier in Europe and the United States, when it was known as consumption, the bacteria literally consuming the body. In this context, the medicine Dr. Vir provided for the workers to give patients was miraculous and brought respect and pride.

The program in Vaishali cured a high proportion of tuberculosis patients—it became a success story. Because at the time many in the country considered Bihar a hopeless backwater, this success was a powerful message: If Bihar could succeed, so could any place in India. What had seemed impossible—effective tuberculosis services throughout the country—now appeared within reach. Success with phased expansion provided the confidence and impetus to expand the program, covering the entire country in just a few years.

After decades analyzing tuberculosis in Europe and Africa, Karel Styblo had created the system Dr. Vir used to treat tuberculosis.[14] This included not only the technical package described in chapter 3 but also his approach to phased expansion. It wasn't a pilot project; pilot projects are the graveyard of innovation. Programs afflicted by "pilot-itis" include those that require intensive training, complex protocols, or extensive resources and might achieve impressive results in a small area but never spread. Styblo didn't speak of pilot projects but of Phase I of systematic expansion. The difference isn't just wording. A pilot project may or may not lead to a broader program (most don't). Phase I presumes and commits to growth. Styblo had three rules for phased expansion. First, implement in at least two places: One area may have idiosyncratic reasons for success or failure. He hedged his bets; Vaishali was one of five Phase I areas in India. Second, choose places with excellent leaders such as Dr. Vir. This maximizes the chance of success and also allows the country to optimize policies as these leaders adapt the policy to the national context. And third, choose places accessible for frequent visits for supportive supervision. Phased expansion allows a country to improve a program during initial implementation so expansion is faster and higher quality.

If a program expands too quickly and quality suffers as a result, the benefits will be far lower than those from careful, phased expansion. But if expansion stalls, many people who could have benefited will suffer avoidable illness or death. Every day of delay may cost lives. Creating and sustaining momentum at the right pace is an art and a science; success is more likely with the phased expansion Styblo taught. Dr. G. R. Khatri, the Indian program director, had to forcefully resist calls for faster expansion—if he hadn't, the program would have cured fewer patients and created more drug-resistant infections.

Phased expansion allows programs to adapt a generic approach to their national context. In the initial phase of the Indian tuberculosis control program, doctors created a "patient-wise box," a shoebox-sized cardboard box containing all medications for one patient's entire treatment.[15] I thought it was a terrible idea. Treatment lasted up to nine months, shipping medicines to health centers took months, and facilities needed to have at least six months' of drug stock available. Because medications expired after two years, these long intervals meant that many drugs would expire and be wasted. What's more, the boxes required lots of space.

The Indian doctors understood, as I did not, that shortages of medication were common and that these shortages undermined tuberculosis control. Most of the times I assumed New York City's experience was relevant to New Delhi, I was wrong. The box ensured that no patient would run out of medications before completing treatment. And, by showing each patient that the full treatment was available at their local health center, the boxes built patients' confidence. The boxes also gave patients a powerful image—the number of pills left in the box showed that completion of their treatment was in sight and strengthened patients' belief they could be cured.[16] (Eventually the regulatory authority extended the approved shelf life of the medications to three years, resolving the drug expiry problem.)

The first phases of a project build optimism and are a time for rapid innovation and change. Ideas that seem great on paper can be ineffective in practice. Creating and rapidly revising prototypes identifies weak points and smooths the way for a scalable package of interventions.[17] Innovation is important to find new routes to progress; it comes in many forms and doesn't necessarily mean creating something new. Often, an innovation adapts or adopts aspects of a program from elsewhere or from other programs. The goal isn't newness—it's effectiveness.

A phased approach allows time to hone technical details and build community, advocacy, and political support. The first phase requires a program to identify which organizations and which parts of government and society can facilitate or block the program, learn to manage these relationships, and find people and organizations who are effective champions for a program. Progress increases the confidence and knowledge of people implementing the project in new areas. Dr. Vir's program in Bihar served as a model for other parts of India: The best-performing areas became training and demonstration sites, proving that success was possible and sharing lessons on how to solve difficult problems.

Recognizing past progress and making more progress through phased expansion—the first two components of the Believe part of the formula—give rational reason for hope. But the most important component is optimism, which isn't just a feel-good emotion, it's a catalyst.

THE POWER OF OPTIMISM

Phased progress can create momentum, but sustaining momentum is hard. Despite a strong start, including in Dr. Vir's district in Bihar, as the Indian tuberculosis program expanded in the late 1990s, it became clear that states, districts, and the national government needed many more staff. The national office oversaw treatment of more than a million patients a year but had only three full-time doctors. It seemed impossible. Dr. Khatri requested approval to hire and train Indian doctors to support the program. The Indian polio eradication initiative had established a similar group of doctors, the model for Khatri's proposal—past progress in another program can show a pathway forward. We raised the funds and prepared for this workforce. The doctors could train health care workers, ensure medicine supply and laboratory quality, get data flowing to track and accelerate progress—basically, be the glue that held the program together.

We were optimistic. Then, the secretary of health, several levels above Khatri in the Ministry of Health hierarchy, rejected the idea. The administrator one level below the secretary saw that the program couldn't succeed without the staff. He recognized that donors would pay the salaries and expenses of the new doctors at no cost to the Government of India. The World Health Organization could hire them, following the example of the polio staff. He understood that they would be transformational and make the government look good. But, shaking his head sadly, he said, "It's not possible." Perhaps one thing about being an American is that it's hard to believe something isn't possible—hard not to be optimistic. Plaintively, I asked if there was a way to solve this problem. He replied, "Dr. Frieden, for some problems, there is no solution."

Dejected, I left the office and asked Khatri to translate—what had the official meant? Obviously it was possible, all it took was one signature. "He is saying," Khatri replied pensively, "that while the current secretary of health remains secretary, it isn't possible. But if he becomes secretary, he'll approve it."

Dr. Fabio Luelmo, who supervised and mentored me in India, taught the importance of patience to preserve optimism. Luelmo, a rail-thin Argentinian who started every day with three cups of coffee, had worked in tuberculosis control programs all over the world and was then based in Geneva with WHO. At one dreary point, progress had stopped, government drug procurement was stuck, health centers were running out of medicine, and I felt like a complete failure. The future looked bleak; I was despondent. Luelmo visited from Geneva, bringing, as usual, a large box of delicious chocolate wafers that would give my family weeks of enjoyment. Luelmo knew how to increase the likelihood that people would be happy to see him. He reviewed my work and told me I was doing great. "But," I protested sincerely, "I've accomplished *nothing*!" "Yes, you have," he replied. "You survived!"

The following year, the Government of India promoted the administrator we had spoken with to the post of secretary and he approved the first group of Indian physicians to support the program. From August of 1999 until today, doctors in these roles have worked at district, state, and national levels in India to improve tuberculosis diagnosis and treatment. When they faced roadblocks, Dr. Khatri provided the political push: He would call the state's health secretary, director general of health, or tuberculosis director to urge, wheedle, cajole, threaten, or order them to make progress. On many occasions, when blocked, he simply caught the next plane to the state capital to negotiate or demand progress. We assigned the doctors to the most challenging districts in the country, yet these districts implemented the program more quickly and with better quality than other districts, demonstrating how important a group of focused, motivated staff can be to the success and scale of a new program.[18] As I was finishing this book, several of the first sixteen of these consultants contacted me—it was the twenty-fifth anniversary of their start, and the group was celebrating their work in India and around the world combating tuberculosis and many other health problems in the years since. The consultants helped cure millions of tuberculosis patients, oversaw training of hundreds of thousands of health care workers, and improved thousands of health centers. Optimism enabled us to get the approvals and to hire, support, and ensure the success of these doctors. Sometimes, optimism required belief in possibilities that defied rational analysis.

IRRATIONAL OPTIMISM

"Irrational optimism," I told the Indian doctors we hired, "is a prerequisite for success." Success—far exceeding what anyone thought possible—required belief that progress was within reach. The polio program not only provided a model for the doctors but achieved the seemingly impossible, vaccinating more than 100 million children in a single campaign.[19] This gave confidence to the public and to doctors, nurses, outreach workers, and others.

Working in another country, it's often essential to keep a low profile, and I did everything I could to stay out of sight in India. I made no statements to the media and gave only one public lecture—a talk at the annual meeting of tuberculosis experts that made the case that tuberculosis can be controlled.[20] Many tuberculosis experts had viewed the disease as one might view the weather: Something to complain about, describe, predict imperfectly, but impossible to control. When it became clear that tuberculosis is not inevitable, progress became feasible.

But just as tuberculosis isn't inevitable, neither is progress. In one massive district in India with a population of more than 10 million, the assigned doctor saw the situation as hopeless. The program had no full-time staff. Many staff were either indifferent or corrupt. Health facilities lacked electricity, water, medications, and staff. A fight among administrators erupted as the state planned to divide the district into several smaller districts, and this fight blocked all progress for more than a year. "But sir," the doctor protested, "sometimes being optimistic goes from irrational to downright illogical!" Several years later, the administrative turmoil subsided, and the program got on track.

Optimism doesn't mean ignoring problems. Progress requires seeing the arc of progress as well as minute and seemingly intractable problems. These two perspectives—big-picture progress and granular difficulties—may appear contradictory, but both can be correct.

On my last night after five years living and working in India, Dr. Khatri hosted a small party. When it was his turn to speak, he said, "Dr. Frieden, the most important thing you did here wasn't all your hard work." This was galling to hear—I had spent years traveling by jeep to most districts of the country, helped write more than 1,000 pages of technical guidance, tracked outcomes every quarter from more than a hundred districts, supervised forty people, and more. I had worked almost every waking hour. "No," he continued. "The most important thing you did here was give us hope."

For individuals, an optimistic attitude correlates with longevity.[21] For programs, it maintains morale, momentum, and a sense of purpose and possibility in the face of inevitable setbacks. Optimistic employees are more proactive and can help persuade politicians to support a program. Despite often-overwhelming challenges, optimism helped recruit, retain, and motivate a great Indian tuberculosis control team.

MISPLACED OPTIMISM

Although optimism is essential for progress, it can be dangerous. For two decades starting in the 1940s, a remarkable public health leader, Fred Soper, known as "The General" although he had no military background, tried to rid the Americas of yellow fever by eliminating the *Aedes aegypti* mosquito.

Tales of the rigor with which Soper pursued the mosquito are legendary.

He would map an area to be cleansed of mosquitoes, give each house a number, and then assign each number to a sector. A sector, in turn, would be assigned to an inspector, armed with the crude pesticides then available; the inspector's schedule for each day was planned to the minute, in advance, and his work double-checked by a supervisor.

If a supervisor found a mosquito that the inspector had missed, he received a bonus. And if the supervisor found that the inspector had deviated by more than ten minutes from his pre-assigned schedule the inspector was docked a day's pay.

Once, in the state of Rio de Janeiro, a large ammunition dump—the Niterói Arsenal—blew up. Soper, it was said, heard the explosion in his office, checked the location of the arsenal on one of his maps, verified by the master schedule that an inspector was at the dump at the time of the accident, and immediately sent condolences and a check to the widow. The next day, the inspector showed up for work, and Soper fired him on the spot—for being alive.[22]

Mosquitoes are hardy species and, despite Herculean efforts, survived in hideouts, buzzing back when Soper's armies were disbanded. Despite this failure, the world launched a global effort to eradicate malaria in the mid-1950s. With DDT spray and antimalarial drugs, the eradication program showed that the world could marshal a massive effort, eliminating malaria from many areas and reducing it in others. The program saved millions of lives, but it failed in its goal of eradication, allowed malaria to come back, and undermined confidence in ambitious public health action. Both programs—mosquito elimination in the Americas and global malaria eradication—failed because they lacked a technical package that could deliver the desired outcome.

Humans have an optimism bias.[23] This bias can be adaptive—improving well-being and leading to experimentation and innovation. But misplaced optimism can be harmful. A common manifestation of the optimism bias is underestimating the time required for a task: Even when experience shows that it takes a long time, we assume we can complete it quickly. This bias may be adaptive—getting us to start a formidable task—and also disruptive, such as when we have to cancel other activities to finish the work. The optimism bias leads us to ignore negative or contradictory information and downplay future risks.[24] This can undermine the response to public health warnings and also reduce the likelihood of carefully considering a public health initiative before undertaking it.

Programs that have unrealistic expectations—such as scaling up a poorly designed initiative or, even if well designed, one without a substantial impact—are examples of misplaced optimism. Misplaced optimism led me to state that any hospital could care for Ebola safely. And I made this mistake with the Million Hearts program, believing we could improve blood pressure control without understanding and changing the underlying economic forces that drive health care in the United States. Unrealistic expectations waste resources and disillusion staff. Programs that overestimate their potential benefit or underestimate the complexities involved set themselves up for failure. They also deny resources to other programs that would have saved lives. For example, programs that focus on screening patients for hypertension without doing the hard work of ensuring that those screened receive appropriate treatment demonstrate misplaced optimism. Screening for hypertension in homes and public places is high-profile and can give impressive numbers—millions of people screened and found with a life-threatening condition. But unless effective treatment programs support patients to start and continue treatment for years, screening does little or no good.[25]

Naïve optimism about what digital innovations, including electronic health records, can achieve has led to billions of dollars being spent poorly.[26] Instead of wasting money on expensive digital systems that help neither patients nor health care workers, countries could have implemented phased digital improvements to expand effective prevention and treatment.

Avoiding misplaced optimism requires understanding whether the interventions will achieve the desired results, whether the capacity to implement these interventions will be created and maintained, and whether the political support for the program will be strong and sustained.

MAINTAINING OPTIMISM

We celebrate success, but it's more productive to celebrate failure. A healthy culture encourages staff to recognize program weaknesses as a prerequisite for improvement. Celebrating failure can prevent repeated mistakes, limit damage, and preserve resources. Celebrating failure preserves the morale of staff who worked hard but, through no fault of their own, didn't achieve the goal. Ironically, "failure festivals" can maintain optimism. Failures are harmful if they cause irreparable damage, result from negligence, or are not openly disclosed and addressed. Failures that cause little or no harm, lead to important learning, and reinforce a culture of continuous improvement can make an initiative or organization stronger.[27]

If the first phase of a program fails, learning what led to the failure fosters creation of a new design. If, later, the program either doesn't scale effectively or stalls during scale-up, analyzing this failure allows a reset and restart that may expand services more effectively. Celebrating failure is a powerful way to use data to improve performance.

An optimistic attitude may seem delusional today with climate change, wars, and bitter divisions in society. Maintaining optimism is particularly important—and may be particularly difficult—for groups that lack economic or political power. Without minimizing or ignoring these realities, it's possible to support the optimistic worldview. Technological advances make work more efficient. Communication platforms make it easier to connect with people around the world. Scientific progress improves our ability to prevent, control, and cure disease with everything from new vaccines to blockbuster drugs. It's important to avoid seeing the past with rose-colored glasses. As Hans Rosling wrote, "Things can be bad and getting better."[28] Bad as things are today, and awful in some parts of the world and for some groups, in the past, slavery, brutality, violence, preventable death and disability, and disenfranchisement of women, racial and ethnic groups, and the poor were far more common. This doesn't excuse continuing injustice or denial of freedoms and opportunities, nor does it diminish the suffering or the urgent need for progress. But it does give important perspective: More progress is possible.

Optimism can be essential—and well-founded—to face problems that may seem intractable, such as improving primary health care. First, recognize past progress. In some ways, good primary care was more common in the past. Decades ago, although far too many Americans couldn't afford it or didn't have access, family doctors—including my father—provided gentle, supportive care. Not only is good primary health care well within reach, it's already here in many places. In the United States today, Kaiser Permanente provides superb primary health care, as do many other integrated systems such as the Mayo Clinic, Cleveland Clinic, Geisinger, and Intermountain Health.[29] Most Scandinavian and many European and Latin American countries provide excellent primary health care. Among middle-income countries, not only Thailand and Costa Rica but also Sri Lanka and Cuba provide reliable primary health care.[30] Next, make phased progress; projects in the United States such as physician-led Accountable Care Organizations demonstrate that more progress is possible.[31]

To shatter the illusion of inevitability, we must—in our own lives and in society—reveal past progress, make additional phased progress, and foster optimism. Optimism motivates action and maintains momentum at all levels—from individuals to health care workers to politicians. But the road to hell is paved with good intentions, and the road to public health failure is paved with naïveté—failure to adapt the science, manage effectively, and navigate politics successfully. To save the most lives, public health must move beyond seeing invisible threats, beyond identifying the pathway to progress, and beyond helping people believe a disaster is avoidable. To protect our own lives, families, and communities, we must succeed at the hardest part of the formula: *Create*.

PART III   CREATE

5 ORGANIZATION

After Bill Foege led the global eradication of smallpox, he was asked what should be done next. He replied, "The eradication of bad management."

An Ebola outbreak in Lagos shows how organization can determine whether we create a healthy future. During a meeting in the CDC emergency operations center in July of 2014, Stuart Nichol, the usually imperturbable lead scientist for the Ebola response, said, with dread in his eyes, "It looks like we have our first case of Ebola in Nigeria, in Lagos." Ebola was raging through Liberia, Sierra Leone, and Guinea but had spared Nigeria. Lagos, the commercial capital of Nigeria, is a chaotic city with more than 20 million people. It has more people and many times more airline flights than the three Ebola-affected countries of West Africa combined. The city also has close ties to northern states of Nigeria, where violence and distrust had made polio eradication particularly challenging.

On July 20, 2014, Patrick Sawyer, a forty-year-old Liberian lawyer, arrived in Lagos and was hospitalized with a high fever. He had refused to believe his Ebola diagnosis in Liberia and didn't tell his Nigerian doctors and nurses about it, leading to a terrifying outbreak. The Nigerian government's initial response wasn't promising. An ineffectual appointee directed the response, and the CDC's lead doctor in Nigeria called the CDC headquarters' emergency operations center in Atlanta, frantic. The previous day, the entire team in charge of stopping the potentially catastrophic outbreak had spent four hours debating what to do about a corpse transiting the country. The individual hadn't died of Ebola or spent time in Liberia—the embalmed corpse had merely passed through that country en route to Nigeria for a traditional funeral. This zero-risk situation consumed nearly all the time of the team in charge of stopping Ebola in Lagos.

While these pointless and interminable discussions continued, doctors and nurses who had been infected with the Ebola virus were dying. Two spent more than twelve hours waiting—in vain—in the back of ambulances for the government to locate a safe isolation facility. Public health workers hadn't notified hundreds of people who had been in contact with Ebola patients; these people could already be spreading the infection. The government wasn't marshaling teams to confront the outbreak, and no isolation facility had been located, much less outfitted, for Ebola care. Ebola is an unforgiving enemy—a single slip can spark an outbreak with hundreds of infections and deaths. The Lagos outbreak could transform the West Africa Ebola epidemic into a global catastrophe that would spread for years and undermine health care in Africa and much of the world. It was the most frightening incident in my years leading the CDC.

Public health is a quintessential government function—all too often undermined by quintessential government incompetence. Because of clunky government bureaucracies, doctors can't do their jobs and patients develop and spread preventable diseases. Even if we see a deadly health threat, understand why we may be reluctant to act, and believe we can stop it, we'll fail unless we act effectively. The first step toward success is to get organized.

INCIDENT MANAGEMENT SYSTEMS

Effective organization can overcome even the most daunting challenge. With calls to leaders in Nigeria, we identified a dynamic Nigerian doctor who had helped stop polio in the country. The Nigerian government put him in charge of the incident management system. Incident management, a system first used to fight forest fires, is a systematic way to manage emergencies by breaking big problems into specific, scalable areas.

Incident management organizes action and allows rapid scale-up of emergency systems. In public health, these areas include surveillance, epidemiology, clinical care, infection prevention and control, contact tracing, training, laboratory services, logistics, research, and communication. Within days, the new leadership team in Lagos trained, organized, and deployed hundreds of staff. They created a practical isolation unit in ten days, trained and supervised staff who visited more than 18,000 contacts of Ebola patients at their homes, and communicated effectively with patients, affected communities, and the media. They stopped the outbreak and prevented a disaster. They then replicated the entire meticulous response in a second city—Port Harcourt, more than 375 miles away—to which two Ebola patients from Lagos had fled. The incident management approach stopped that outbreak also.[1] Stopping Ebola in Lagos prevented deaths not just from Ebola but also from disruption of life-saving health services such as vaccination programs and malaria treatment.

When Nigeria implemented an incident management system to manage the Ebola outbreak, they pivoted from ineffectual response to complete control. In tragic contrast, lack of effective organization in the US effort to confront the COVID pandemic in 2020 was deadly. The Trump administration didn't take the first step of emergency response—establish an incident management system to develop, communicate, and implement policy. Many entities seemed to be in charge, and, as is common when this happens, none was.

Faced with the biggest infectious disease crisis in a century, throughout 2020, the US wasn't even organized for battle. A competent administration would have created a clear strategy and structure to fight the virus, with empowered incident managers aligned with political leaders at national, state, and local levels. This would have enabled systematic testing, hospitalization, isolation, contact tracing, and quarantine. It would have provided daily briefings with accurate and timely information and guidance from credible, nonpolitical physicians not associated with any elected official. It would have protected health care workers and enabled health care systems to safely treat COVID patients and those who needed health care not related to COVID. It would have modulated business closures to protect both the economy and health. It would have supported the nutritional, educational, health, and financial needs of people in isolation or quarantine. A competent, organized response would have engaged communities, obtained information through surveys, assessed adherence to masking and other recommendations, and used findings to save lives and reduce disruption. Although some cities and states had effective responses, and although many other countries implemented most or all of these measures, not a single one of these fundamentally important actions occurred nationally in the US in 2020.

Asked about the absence of incident management, President Trump and Vice President Pence stated that Pete Gaynor, the administrator of the Federal Emergency Management Agency (FEMA), was in charge.[2] Was Gaynor, with no public health experience, raising policy issues for the White House to decide? What was the role of Jared Kushner, the president's son-in-law? Was FEMA supervising the Coronavirus Task Force that the vice president chaired? How did Secretary of Health and Human Services Alex Azar and his agencies, including the CDC, relate to Gaynor? What was the role of Dr. Tony Fauci, director of the National Institute of Allergy and Infectious Diseases? President Trump had appointed Dr. Deborah Birx White House coronavirus response coordinator. What was her role? This lack of clarity violated the fundamental rule of organization in an emergency.

Since its establishment in 1946, the CDC had been central to the US response to every health emergency. In contrast, during 2020, as the COVID pandemic killed hundreds of thousands of Americans, the CDC was neither at the table providing information so decisions could balance health and other considerations nor at the podium explaining them.

When, months later, FEMA went back to its usual work responding to hurricanes and other emergencies, organization and management remained astonishingly unclear. In a coherent response, the federal government sets specific, practical guidance and provides resources, oversight, and technical assistance. States and cities then adapt and implement this guidance, making it appropriate for their communities. During the first year of the COVID pandemic, guidance from the federal government was late, incomplete, and sometimes inappropriate.

By February 2020, Resolve to Save Lives had helped more than a dozen countries in Africa create, strengthen, or activate an emergency management system for COVID. It was horrifying to see the United States lack even a minimally competent incident management structure, with no systematic approach to operations, supplies, or information.

Future threats—ranging from new microbes to climate impacts—will require organized, flexible responses. Success will also require prioritization.

PRIORITIZATION

Incident management systems help during emergencies, but are just one way to organize for progress and save lives in the Create part of the See/Believe/Create formula. An incident management system forces and facilitates prioritization, a difficult concept for many political leaders to accept. Even when there's no emergency, prioritizing is hard. One path to progress is to focus on important, nonurgent issues. Urgent issues—an outbreak, a public outcry, a political initiative—demand attention. A flood of requirements, meetings, document requests, and urgent—or supposedly urgent—projects often trap people in reactive mode. Breaking this pattern requires focus.

Stephen Covey popularized an approach of President Dwight Eisenhower.[3] In the top left of a 2×2 table, quadrant I, are urgent and important activities such as investigating a potentially deadly outbreak (table 5.1). In quadrant II, at the top right, are initiatives that are important but not urgent, such as advocating for a tobacco tax or improving a disease tracking system. Quadrant III at the bottom left includes tasks that are urgent but not important (that memo the boss wants immediately for a meeting on an unimportant topic and which will likely go unread). Quadrant IV at the bottom right contains emails, news trackers, and other work that is neither urgent nor important. The natural tendency is to spend most time working in quadrants I, III, and IV. Increasing the time spent on quadrant II projects creates a virtuous cycle, with fewer urgent requests and less low-productivity work.

Applying the matrix to hypertension makes the approach clear. Although hospitals provide urgent care for people with heart attacks and strokes (quadrant I), improving blood pressure control through better diagnosis, treatment, and information systems (quadrant II) can prevent these emergencies.[4] Progress in quadrant II reduces the need to spend time in quadrant I and can save more lives.

Table 5.1

Matrix to manage public health time and resources

	Urgent	Not urgent
Important	*Quadrant I* Respond to suspected disease outbreak Respond to a natural disaster Address shortages in medical supplies during an epidemic Provide clinical guidance for an emerging health threat Respond to urgent question or request from a political leader	*Quadrant II* Build a coalition to advocate for change, including stronger connections with clinical and other sectors Mentor staff and create a leadership development program Improve laws, technologies, and procedures to prevent or better manage outbreaks, including better information systems, vaccination, sanitation, and early detection and treatment Improve financial sustainability Change policies so there is less risk of development and spread of disease
Not Important	*Quadrant III* Emails, avoidable paperwork, and requests for calls, meetings, presentations Meetings attended by too many people, poorly organized, with limited potential for impact Declarations and calls for action without practical means to achieve progress Deadlines looming because of insufficient planning or artificial milestones and timelines Responding to media requests that don't lead to accurate or useful coverage	*Quadrant IV* Tracking news and social media without a specific focus or limit Nonstrategic networking activities Social media debates unlikely to advance health Webinars or other events that have limited relevance and with information that can be absorbed more efficiently by other means Mandatory training of limited utility

A 2 × 2 table divides issues into four quadrants. Focusing on quadrant II—important, nonurgent issues—enables a proactive agenda protecting and promoting health rather than reacting to daily crises.

But progress becomes possible only when organizations implement a classic quadrant II activity—creating and supporting great teams.

TEAMS

In the early 1990s, New York City faced the deadly high-profile crisis of multidrug-resistant tuberculosis that Karen Brudney had recognized. The unit fighting the outbreak was understaffed and demoralized, with poor performance, dilapidated clinics, and little connection to the doctors treating patients. Dr. Brudney was scathing: In public lectures, she called my bumbling predecessor as head of the New York City tuberculosis contro program a "war criminal." Even after we saw the outbreak, believed it could be stopped, and designed an effective technical approach, we would fail without an effective team.

Karen Brudney had revealed the invisible—the dramatic and previously unrecognized increase in drug resistance. Karel Styblo's technical package showed the way forward and demonstrated that progress was possible. This fulfilled the See and Believe parts of the formula. But to succeed—to Create a solution and prevent tuberculosis—required managing a crisis despite a sleepy government bureaucracy. How would this be possible? Fresh from Epidemic Intelligence Service training and in my first management role, I had no idea.

Public services face harsh criticism as slow, ineffectual, and wasteful—real problems that reflect the constraints on public sector management. Hiring, purchasing, and contracting follow cumbersome processes designed more to avoid scandal than achieve outcomes. Health problems seem inevitable. Administrative leaders don't share a sense of urgency. Elected leaders rarely have political incentives for public health action. Budgets are insufficient. Administration is too rigid to allow innovation. Information systems seldom show whether programs are succeeding or failing.

The CDC sent Louis Salinas, a superb operational expert, to coach me. Salinas was brutally honest. In a series of single-spaced letters over the course of a year, amid some (very) faint praise, he informed me that staff

> feel extremely reluctant to question or challenge you. . . . The following are adjectives I've heard to describe you . . . impatient . . . inexperienced . . . micromanager . . . poor communicator . . . unfocused. . . . You act as if, if not for the limits of time and space, you would do every job yourself. You may work twice as many hours and three times as fast as others, but what six people do in an organization of 600 people isn't very important.

Salinas taught me to build a team; strengthen systems; find and motivate superb staff; fix purchasing and contracting; support outreach workers, doctors, and nurses; and get the right messages to medical staff, hospital administrators, budget offices, the mayor, and the press. The tuberculosis control program needed to go from an underperforming to an excellent

to make progress if they implement three principles for institutional success: *mission, pragmatism*, and *effective use of data*. Mission is essential: It allows leaders and staff to focus on activities with the greatest impact.[8] A strong sense of mission helps recruit and retain excellent staff and build morale. The most effective organizations provide their staff with a sense of meaning—that their work has value.

The second essential principle—pragmatism—requires tight connection with the realities of the people served. The secret sauce of CDC's success in smallpox eradication and other programs has been pairing an epidemiologist with a public health advisor—someone like Louis Salinas, who gave me such blunt feedback. Epidemiologists may know *what* to do; public health advisors are more likely to know *how* to get it done. An epidemiologist might know that controlling an outbreak requires a vaccination campaign in a particular community. A public health advisor can find the people, places, and equipment needed to make the campaign happen—and manage all the details of implementing the campaign.[9]

A rotation system is one way to solidify this pragmatic approach, with staff alternating between local work and headquarters, starting with a multi-year stint in a local organization. This isn't a new idea. Dr. Joseph Mountin, who created the CDC, wanted staff to first spend a year as a county health officer—long enough to propose a budget and get it approved.[10] Professionals would then better understand how to design and adapt programs. If pragmatism permeates an organization, when headquarters makes a recommendation, people whose job is to implement the recommendation are less likely to roll their eyes because of an obvious disconnect with what's possible. To remain effective as populations age and become more diverse, organizations will need to adapt their services, staffing, and priorities.

Using data for management is the third essential component of effective organizations. In the private sector, the market provides an essential feedback loop—if people don't like a product, it doesn't sell. When a government agency implements a program that doesn't work, no mechanism prevents the program from continuing indefinitely. Similarly, a nonprofit organization may continue activities for as long as it receives funds; effective programs may stop because of lack of money and ineffective programs may continue despite achieving little. Institutions must create feedback loops to enable rapid course corrections. The New York City community health survey showed that progress reducing smoking had stalled; without that information, we wouldn't have gotten back on track. As discussed in chapter 1, the public health superpower of surveillance also applies to program monitoring—the best programs have inbuilt, timely tracking systems to determine whether they're off course.

When New York City launched a two-week program to give nicotine patches to smokers who wanted to quit, we used real-time tracking to increase the impact of the effort. Smokers could call 311, the city's information line, to request the patches, and we tracked recipients by zip code. Data from the community survey made smoking rates in each community visible, enabling us to calculate, for each neighborhood, what proportion of smokers had called. Each evening, the health department analyzed the data, and the next day sent college students to the neighborhoods with lower participation rates to distribute leaflets encouraging smokers to call for the free medication and to quit smoking.

Some management challenges are complex, but some solutions are simple. On my first day of internship, the senior resident instructed: "Make a list of the things you need to do each day. Throughout the day, cross them off as you do them. If you're going to call your mother because it's her birthday, write it down. If you can't get something done and it can wait, make the next day's list with it on top. When you've crossed everything off the list, you can go home." Stunningly simple, rarely done, enormously helpful, and beautifully described in Atul Gawande's book *The Checklist Manifesto: How to Get Things Right*.[11]

Organization—crucial to create a healthier future—requires structure, prioritization, and stronger institutions. Well-functioning institutions make it easier to implement programs. But although the "only people matter" view is wrong, institutions must have effective staff.

HIRING

In 1991, Karen Brudney's insight and the CDC lab results made it clear that multidrug-resistant tuberculosis was spreading throughout the city.

During my first Health Department cabinet meeting—chaired by the commissioner and attended by all senior leaders—I described the crisis: Patients were spreading tuberculosis and dying. Although we had funds to bring on hundreds of urgently needed staff, bureaucratic inflexibility blocked every hire. As I talked, I got angrier and angrier, then stormed out of the wood-paneled office to go to clinic, saying I had desperately ill patients waiting. It was the last cabinet meeting I was invited to.

Puzzling over how to accelerate hiring after leaving the meeting, I remembered my EIS training and applied the concept of surveillance to the hiring process. Each week, our program sent charts to the commissioner and her administrative chief showing the timeliness of the twenty-seven steps it took to hire a single employee. The data revealed two major bottlenecks. First, the city's budget office took many months to approve each person we proposed to hire. Although they eventually approved every request, by the time they did so, many applicants had found other jobs. By changing the system so they reviewed each staff member hired *after* the person started and, if necessary, adjusted salary or terminated employment, we reduced the median time for this process from 117 days to zero. (Whether the budget office should review every résumé of every person hired in city government is a good question. It was easier to change the process than eliminate it. Commissioner Margaret "Peggy" Hamburg often reminded me not to let the perfect be the enemy of the good.)

The second bottleneck was the need for physical examinations by the department's employee health program before candidates could start work. The plodding physician who ran the program explained that, even with more resources, he and his team couldn't possibly do more than twenty-five physical examinations a week. There were nearly 1,000 staff, including 400 for the tuberculosis control program, who would need examinations. This meant a months- or years-long delay. With five other physicians from the tuberculosis control program, we took over the employee health center on Saturdays, each of us conducting ten to fifteen physical examinations a day, and cleared the backlog in a few weeks.

The hiring process was not only slow, but also fundamentally flawed. An evocative 1948 memoir of a patient with tuberculosis described our dingy clinics well, half a century later:

The [Tuberculosis] Clinic shared a building with the police station, city jail, emergency hospital, and venereal disease clinic. The dark, ancient elevator seemed to have caught some virulent ailment from its patients for, when it was loaded, it coughed and wheezed, lost its breath entirely, dropped back a foot or two, bounced uncertainly for awhile and finally by summoning up every ounce of its strength managed to struggle up to the second floor. . . . The clinic was a depressing place filled with golden oak benches, stale air and other people with TB.[12]

The doctors in the clinics were even more problematic than the dilapidated buildings. Two retired pathologists had never treated live patients previously. Another doctor, in his mid-eighties, had retired from clinical practice after becoming completely deaf. He didn't read lips, his handwriting was illegible, and he didn't use a computer, making communication to and from patients cumbersome or impossible. One doctor made bizarre and meandering statements that had led prior employers to fire him. What's more, the low pay made it unlikely their replacements would be much better. To improve the clinics—and stop the tuberculosis outbreak—we needed better doctors. We had to increase salaries. Even seeing the problems, believing in progress, and getting organized wouldn't help without the right people in the right jobs.

Increasing salaries isn't easy. Many people view government salaries as too high. Nongovernmental organizations also grapple with the belief that their staff salaries should be low. The political economy of government jobs favors large numbers of low-paid staff—providing opportunities for patronage or, at least, support for constituent jobs. Skilled professionals in government generally earn far less than their counterparts in the private sector.[13] Care of multidrug-resistant tuberculosis was as complex as cancer chemotherapy, with potentially toxic medications that required expert clinical management. With hundreds of patients needing treatment, we urgently needed highly skilled doctors. But how could we get them?

Enter Lenny. Lenny was in charge of creating new job titles in New York City government. He had been in that position for decades, and people throughout city government feared and respected him. During meetings over several weeks, he noted that the public hospitals organization had a title for specialized physicians, known informally as "superdoc"; the salary would be high enough to hire competent physicians. One pathway to progress is to base proposals on analogous existing programs, as the tuberculosis consultants in India had been based on the successful polio eradication staff. Lenny approved the medical subspecialist title with a higher pay scale. We hired excellent physicians who provided the required complex care. Sadly, Lenny died the following year. We had hired new doctors with the superdoc title, but Lenny hadn't formalized it. That title became known as "Dead Lenny's Title"; all formal approvals were issued years later. Analogous to the superdoc title, the CDC and other federal agencies use the "Distinguished Scientist" title to pay competitive salaries to the highly skilled doctors and other specialists needed to address complex health problems.

To recruit additional competent physicians and train the next generation of tuberculosis leaders, we began a program for specialists-in-training. The trainees provided good care to hundreds of patients and learned the intricacies of tuberculosis clinical treatment. The training program also upgraded the tuberculosis control program: Supervisors had to systematize protocols, answer trainees' challenging questions, and analyze their own data. Trainees can force an organization to improve.

Similarly, the Epidemic Intelligence Service training program forced the CDC to become a better institution. Supervisors needed to know and teach advanced skills in epidemiology, biostatistics, and scientific writing. Program managers needed good relations with state and local health departments. That way, CDC could post staff to these departments for two years, as they had posted me to New York City. The media office had to explain fast-evolving outbreaks. Laboratories needed to solve infectious disease and other health mysteries. And all of this required the CDC to be available 24/7, every day of the year.

In addition to highly trained physicians, we needed outreach workers who could relate well to tuberculosis patients. This meant staff who were able to connect with homeless patients, who spoke the languages of patients from other countries, and who could earn the trust of patients who were deeply suspicious of government. Health organizations need staff with a broad range of skills, from epidemiology to law, regulation, communication, informatics, advocacy, and more. Building diverse teams that reflect the communities they serve isn't just about fairness, it's also essential for effectiveness.

The most effective way to recruit superb staff is the same as one of the essentials of an effective organization: a strong sense of mission. The motto of the Johns Hopkins Bloomberg School of Public Health applies to the entire field: *Saving Lives, Millions at a Time*. Well-performing health programs are run by teams that have a strong sense of camaraderie. Rather than "work-life balance"—which may imply a seesaw, with the good parts of life weighed down by drudgery at work—a better concept is a balanced life that includes meaningful and satisfying work and loving and supportive home relationships and friendships. This reflects the classic definition of mental health attributed to Sigmund Freud: "To love and to work."

But even after implementing the See and Believe parts of the formula and even after starting to Create by getting organized, prioritizing, strengthening organizations, and hiring great staff, there's a lurking danger that can undermine progress. Even the best staff can't succeed in a corrupt system.

THE CORROSION OF CORRUPTION

It simply was not done. In 1995, the head of WHO's tuberculosis control program wrote to India's secretary of health conveying his alarm at the "ill-advised" decision to purchase a large quantity of anti-tuberculosis drugs to be given to patients without careful monitoring. The phrase "ill-advised" was an inspired word choice; it enabled the secretary to avoid blame. If the government went through with the purchase, which would provide a kickback to the doctor who arranged it, hundreds of thousands of patients would receive incomplete treatment with the most effective anti-tuberculosis drug—and thousands would soon harbor and spread strains of tuberculosis resistant to this drug. Tuberculosis could become untreatable in India and beyond. In response to this blunt, unprecedented letter, the Indian government halted the purchase and looked for another doctor to replace the corrupt one who had placed the order.

Meanwhile, Dr. G. R. Khatri was quietly sipping whiskey and soda in a remote, violent village in the Indian state of West Bengal. Several years before the letter from WHO, Khatri had been one of the most prominent doctors in the country, in the important position of overseeing health at the ports. His boss had asked him, in a meeting with fifteen other top government doctors, to sign a form attesting that expensive medical equipment being imported tax-free was for charitable organizations. It wasn't: A corrupt group would resell the equipment to for-profit hospitals, avoiding a large import tax. The money saved by tax evasion would provide a hefty illegal payoff to the government doctors. "Dr. Khatri," the director general of health services said, "you must sign the form." "I won't sign it," Dr. Khatri replied evenly, "because you are a corrupt bastard." The next morning, Khatri was transferred to the remote field station. (Many years later when I mentioned this, he laughed and said, "Oh, that was the third or fourth time I was thrown out, always for the same reason!") After canceling the corrupt procurement, the health secretary looked for someone honest to run the program, plucked Khatri out of West Bengal, and put him in charge. Khatri restarted the program and implemented it effectively.

Past corruption or alleged corruption has scarred public sector administrative systems. It was the major reason hiring a single employee in New York City required twenty-seven separate steps. The larger loss of public dollars is often from inefficiency, not corruption.[14]

We shouldn't smugly think corruption is limited to lower-income countries. Years after I left India, Dr. Khatri called me. Dejected about another corruption incident, he asked, "Dr. Frieden, do you have corruption in your country?" "Well," I replied, "in our country, if a company gives money to a politician and the politician gets a law passed that benefits the company, it's legal." Recent events in the US show the importance of safeguards and transparency in public hiring, contracting, budgeting, and procurement.

Corruption undermines governance and economic growth, exacerbates inequality, and blocks public health action. The See/Believe/Create formula applies to stopping corruption: See the costs of corruption, the benefits of preventing it, and the path to progress. Singapore, Estonia, and other countries have reduced corruption—giving confidence in the integrity of public services in these places and in the possibility of progress elsewhere. Successful programs work with administrators to build corruption-resistant, efficient systems that reduce the number of steps and approvals needed and increase the transparency of interactions and timelines. These programs track perceptions of corruption, improve hiring and promotion, disseminate clear ethical guidelines, and instill pride in good performance. They establish independent commissions, public reporting hotlines, and websites, with accountability for follow-up; use data mining and forensic analysis to identify possible corruption; protect journalists and whistleblowers; and engage reform-minded public servants and effective nongovernmental organizations such as Transparency International. Despite substantial odds, vibrant civil society, coupled with rigorous, specific action, can lead to steady progress.[15]

Civil society organizations can help fight corruption, but they can also do much more.

NONGOVERNMENTAL ORGANIZATIONS AND THE FORMULA

Nongovernmental organizations can drive progress implementing all parts of the formula. They sound alarms to see the invisible, build confidence that progress is possible, and implement policies and programs.

In June of 2014, Dr. Joanne Liu was outraged. She was international president of Médecins Sans Frontières. As Ebola spread out of control in West Africa, her treatment centers were stretched to the limit and had to turn patients away. She and her staff had warned global leaders for months and were now experiencing an exponential increase in Ebola cases. When cases exploded in Monrovia, Liberia, she sounded an alarm: Urban Ebola was different.[16] Initially, CDC staff thought she was wrong: The Ebola virus doesn't change in urban areas. But she was right. In rural areas, one patient might expose family members and a few others. In crowded urban areas, infectious patients seeking care exposed dozens of people at home and often took multiple taxi and motorcycle rides to hospitals. Dr. Liu sounded the alarm that helped trigger more intensive action to stop the Ebola epidemic. She knew what was happening because 90 percent of MSF staff treating patients were from the affected communities and they told her what was happening—MSF had the essential pragmatic connection with reality. And she wasn't afraid to speak up because MSF's broad funding base gave them independence. They didn't hesitate to make the invisible visible so the world would see the epidemic.

Resolve to Save Lives has advanced the Believe part of the formula, building confidence that hypertension can be controlled. In low- and middle-income countries, few health centers treated hypertension: It was seen as either too complicated, too expensive, or not relevant. The condition affects approximately one third of adults; huge numbers of patients need treatment. Many clinics lack the staff, medications, and information systems necessary for lifelong care of people with hypertension. Strokes and heart attacks from untreated hypertension seemed inevitable.

Using Styblo's approach of a technical package—HEARTS, described in chapter 3—and his strategy of phased implementation to build confidence described in chapter 4, Resolve to Save Lives partners with dozens of countries to establish policies, protocols, staff, equipment, medications, and information systems. This demonstrates to doctors, nurses, and country leaders that what seemed hopeless—treating hypertension to prevent heart attacks and strokes—is within reach. But sometimes seeing and believing isn't enough—only a political push can make the Create part of the formula possible.

The Carter Center builds coalitions to stop devastating but neglected diseases, advocating for people who lack political power. Guinea worm disease causes such severe pain it's known as "fiery serpent disease." In the 1980s, an estimated 3.5 million people became infected each year. The Carter Center has prevented 80 million people from getting the disease through its support for mass drug administration, health education, and community mobilization. Guinea worm is now close to eradication. The Center's success in the Create part of the formula stems in large part from its ability to bridge the political and the public health realms through President Jimmy Carter's credibility. He met with heads of state in affected countries, transcended political and social divides, and convinced leaders to see and address diseases the world had long ignored.[17]

All organizations face difficulties maintaining the three essential principles for organizational success: mission, pragmatism, and data-driven progress. Receiving government funds may compromise an organization's mission and consume staff and leadership time. One group that has maintained focus is the Drugs for Neglected Diseases initiative (DNDi). Their mission is crystal clear: the best science for the most neglected diseases. Since 2003, DNDi has developed thirteen treatments for six infections, including drugs for deadly and disabling diseases such as malaria, leishmaniasis, Chagas disease, and sleeping sickness. These innovations have given millions of people longer, healthier lives.[18] The organization stays focused on rigorous science to develop new treatments for neglected diseases, turning down funding for other projects, such as those to develop treatments for other diseases.

As organizations grow, they risk becoming inefficient—of losing their pragmatism. MSF has largely avoided this. The organization cares for people affected by conflict, epidemics, and disasters in more than seventy countries. Although no organization is perfect, MSF remains nimble despite its large operations. It reviews what it's accomplishing with each project and has a structured, disciplined way to end missions. It closes some of its projects every year, allowing it to respond to emerging needs. MSF's financial independence makes this possible. Millions of individual donors provide flexible funds so MSF can respond without having to fundraise first, and this independence also shields it from political pressures. MSF has grown rapidly and has a budget of nearly $2 billion per year, larger than many international agencies. MSF limits spending on headquarters and administration to 20 percent of its total, forcing it to spend 80 percent on field operations.

In India, the Aravind Eye Care System uses data and innovation—the third principle of effective organizations—in the Create part of the formula. Optimizing every aspect of cataract surgery and rigorously assessing the outcomes of their patients, they perform millions of surgeries and manufacture ophthalmic products, providing high quality at costs that can be 100 times lower than in high-income countries. Aravind was an early adopter of telemedicine, reaching hundreds of thousands of people who would otherwise not receive care. With this approach, Aravind has been able to deliver superb eye care to millions of people.

Organization can help people see, believe, and act to prevent future tragedies. But to make rapid progress in the Create aspect of the See/Believe/Create formula, simplicity is essential.

6 SIMPLE, SCALABLE SOLUTIONS

Simplicity is the ultimate sophistication.
—Leonardo da Vinci

Dr. Karel Styblo's question was straightforward: "Of the 3,811 patients with tuberculosis diagnosed in New York City last year, how many did you cure?" I didn't know, and was deeply ashamed.

It was January of 1993, half a year after I became head of the New York City tuberculosis control program. Styblo explained, "Tuberculosis control is really very simple. Just one rule: No cheating. Every patient in your area, you are responsible for their outcome." Styblo's question changed the way I have thought and worked ever since. Styblo understood how tuberculosis spreads—explaining R_0 to me on the back of a napkin—and established a technical package to control the disease, described in chapter 3. He had shown how to build confidence through phased expansion, discussed in chapter 4. But Styblo's laser-like focus on outcomes—on how to save the most lives—underpinned all of these insights: He saw that the most important fact is not the *number* but the *proportion* of all patients cured. Most programs miss that obvious but essential information in a blizzard of data. Successful health programs use simple approaches that expand quickly to reach everyone in need—simplicity, speed, and scale, a life-saving triad in the *Create* part of the formula.

THE SIMPLE TRUTH

This simple truth—the outcome of every patient, no excuses—transformed tuberculosis control. This truth is an example of a broader approach essential to scale up programs and save lives: simplicity. Even with a clear understanding of how tuberculosis spreads and how to stop it (See), optimism from past progress and phased expansion (Believe), and a well-organized, well-staffed program, success requires a simple, practical approach.

Dr. Karen Brudney worked with Styblo on tuberculosis control in Central America. Styblo gave her a blank register with columns for patient name, dates of diagnosis and treatment, lab tests, and whether and when the patient completed treatment. He called her from his office in the Netherlands to review every patient whose outcome was missing from the register and check the proportion of patients who completed treatment. Styblo's approach is to perform an unforgiving prospective cohort analysis—monitoring the outcome of every person diagnosed.

When Brudney moved back to the United States in 1988, during New York City's tuberculosis resurgence, she analyzed all patients diagnosed with tuberculosis at Harlem Hospital. Using Styblo's method, she tracked patients after hospital discharge and found that the program cured only 11 percent—the rest were either lost to follow-up or dead.[1] The Styblo approach is, for many health problems, the only accurate way to determine and improve quality. It's a simple concept: Every program is responsible for every patient diagnosed in its area, no exceptions. This approach is foreign to doctors, nurses, hospital administrators, and political leaders, who focus on the patient or voter in front of them, not the actual outcomes of all people in need, which is the proportion of the total, not the number. Clinicians may be oblivious to the patients who have stopped treatment or never started it. Prospective cohort evaluation—a simple approach to make the invisible visible—holds a key to improve health care.

The day after Styblo's visit, we began reviews of every cohort of patients, in every part of the city, every quarter. Initially, patient after patient had been lost to follow-up. I left those reviews nearly in tears, as did other leaders and staff—it seemed hopeless. But then teams did whatever it took to get treatment to patients. Outreach workers went to park benches, homeless encampments, abandoned buildings—anywhere to help patients with their social needs and give them treatment. These were the frontline heroes who reversed the tuberculosis epidemic. And now the answer to Styblo's question is that, from far less than half when he visited, New York City has for many years cured nearly all tuberculosis patients.

Cohort reviews revealed many problems, ranging from outreach workers needing cars so they could visit patients who lived far from public transport, to overcrowded clinics where staff treated patients rudely, to private doctors who prescribed the wrong medications. Solutions to these problems were sometimes complex, but the bottom line was simple: Every patient. No exceptions. Reviewing every patient forced the program to address each problem systematically. At the next quarterly review, we would see if our solution had worked. If it had, we congratulated and encouraged staff. If it hadn't, we looked for new ways to solve hard problems.

Dr. Fabio Luelmo, the supervisor who encouraged me in India, had worked with Styblo and commented that, as cerebral as Styblo's approach was, when he spoke with patients, he demonstrated deep caring. Focusing on outcomes doesn't mean ignoring individual patients but rather working to ensure that the program doesn't ignore even a single patient. Equity—reaching everyone, especially those most likely to be neglected—is a core philosophy of public health, not only because it's ethically right but also because it's essential to control disease.

In a meeting at the World Health Organization in Geneva to establish an evaluation system, others proposed a long list of complex indicators to measure what was done, by whom, how many times. These were process indicators, cumbersome to collect and rarely resulting in improved patient care. Luelmo insisted that the focus be the cure rate; health centers could choose to track additional, detailed information to improve the cure rate. As he walked out of this contentious meeting with another participant, she sneered what she thought was an insult at him: "Oh, you're one of those *outcome* people."

For the Create part of the See/Believe/Create formula, effective organization, discussed in chapter 5, is essential. But even the best-organized efforts fail without a strategic approach to implementation, starting with simplicity. Simplicity, with an approach such as Styblo's unforgiving cohort evaluation, is essential because only simple approaches are likely to be implementable at scale.

SIMPLICITY IN DIAGNOSIS, TREATMENT, AND MONITORING

Styblo's simple approach to tuberculosis can also transform the treatment of hypertension. At most 20 percent of people in the world with hypertension have it under control. Every year, among the more than one billion people with high blood pressure, there are more than 10 million deaths and tens of millions more nonfatal heart attacks and strokes. Many of these occur among people in their forties and fifties. Untreated and undertreated hypertension also leads to kidney failure and dementia. Simplification is essential to make progress stopping what has become the world's leading killer.

Working with WHO and others, Resolve to Save Lives adapted Styblo's tuberculosis approach to high blood pressure—the technical package outlined in chapter 3. Previously, the approach for patients with elevated blood pressure had been to advise them to lose weight, eat healthier food, increase physical activity, and come back in three months. Most patients didn't return, and of those who did, very few changed their habits sufficiently to reduce blood pressure. Programs almost never analyzed what actually happened to the patients they had advised to change their habits and come back—the basic Styblo question. In fact, hardly any came back with their blood pressure controlled. To improve outcomes, simplicity was essential. A simple policy, now used in more than forty countries, requires just two blood pressure readings before treatment: same-day for very high pressure, different days for moderately high. This increases the number of patients treated—and therefore the number of heart attacks, strokes, and deaths prevented.[2]

And that's just the process to decide *which* patients to treat. Deciding *how* to treat them has also often been far too complex. Reminiscent of President Eisenhower's criticism of a political opponent as being so smart he can see eleven sides to every two-sided question, guidance has included multiple medication and dosage choices. In contrast, an effective, simple algorithm chosen by local or national providers takes a structured, linear approach based on a single data point—blood pressure. Figure 6.1 shows one such protocol, which uses just four steps and can control blood pressure in more than 80 percent of patients.[3] As varied as patients are, a simple

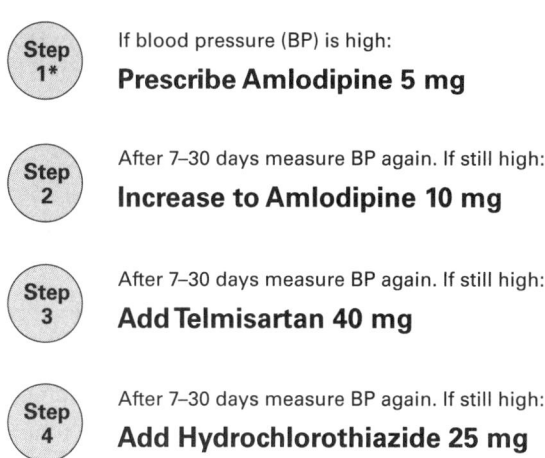

Step 1* — If blood pressure (BP) is high:
Prescribe Amlodipine 5 mg

Step 2 — After 7–30 days measure BP again. If still high:
Increase to Amlodipine 10 mg

Step 3 — After 7–30 days measure BP again. If still high:
Add Telmisartan 40 mg

Step 4 — After 7–30 days measure BP again. If still high:
Add Hydrochlorothiazide 25 mg

*If blood pressure is ≥160/100, begin at Step 2.
For frail elderly patients, begin at Amlodipine 2.5 mg.

Figure 6.1

A four-step algorithm to treat patients with hypertension. A linear treatment algorithm is more likely to be adhered to than one with branches. The fewer steps, the more likely clinicians will follow them. Simple algorithms enable more patients to be treated effectively in more clinical settings.

protocol using just three medications works well. Selecting an algorithm requires understanding thousands of scientific articles on the safety, efficacy, and interactions of medications. It also requires practical understanding of whether and which laboratory tests are needed and the availability and cost of these tests and of the medications. A simple approach sees complex reality and develops a practical solution to change it.

Simple algorithms make it possible to train staff better, purchase quality-assured medications for less money, reduce the risk of running out of drugs, and enable more members of the health care team to help patients. When different treatment is indicated—for example, for patients with hypertension and kidney failure—a different approach is used. Clinicians can depart from the standard approach if they feel this is clinically indicated, although those who do so often find that their control rates are lower than those of clinicians who follow the algorithm.

Simplicity is particularly important for information systems. Simpler systems are more likely to be used, up-to-date, and accurate. In an emergency, only simple systems can be scaled up. In many countries, essential surveillance data, ranging from infectious disease case numbers to immunization rates to records of births and deaths are incomplete and inaccurate. A major reason for information gaps is avoidable complexity. It seems obvious, but remains controversial: To improve hypertension control, it's essential to track the number and proportion of patients with their blood pressure controlled. This approach can more than double control rates.[4]

Styblo created a wonderful information system for tuberculosis, simple and easy even for health care workers with little training and minimal literacy. The system made data falsification easy to spot and facilitates rapid improvement. Although paper-based records work for tuberculosis, there are at least fifty times more patients with hypertension, so a digital system is needed. Hypertension treatment programs now use the Styblo concept to steadily increase the proportion of patients with controlled blood pressure. Our team created an app called Simple, which enables health care workers to record information accurately during the patient's visit. Although smart and dedicated leaders create digital systems they believe will work, it's essential to see what happens when busy health care workers in clinics with limited internet connectivity try to use it. Health care workers could collect lots of data at each visit, but in many countries they have less than five minutes per patient—time better spent listening to and speaking with patients than entering data. Digital tools must replace paper or data will be incomplete and inaccurate.

Our team reduced the time needed to enter data for follow-up visits to an average of thirteen seconds. That was fast enough for health care workers to stop using paper records.[5] The app saves nurses, on average, twenty-four minutes every day.[6] Reports that previously took two to three hours to calculate now require just two to three taps on a smartphone screen or clicks on a computer. With this approach, programs can treat more patients and treat them more effectively. Achieving this level of simplicity required constantly reevaluating what actually happened when nurses entered data, trying different approaches, and optimizing the software. The concepts from the Simple app have now been embedded into multiple other digital systems.

Achieving simplicity is the first step toward implementing successfully—but only the first step. Once there's a simple approach based on sound science, speed becomes essential—the faster we act, the more lives we can save.

SPEED

Patience doesn't come naturally to me. In 1992, when I became director of New York City's tuberculosis control program, my executive assistant gave me a Post-it pad that said, "No rush. An hour ago is fine." Dr. Martin Luther King Jr. said it best: We must feel "the fierce urgency of now." But even after decades of public health work, I didn't grasp just how important speed is until my first trip to the epicenter of the Ebola epidemic.

In August of 2014, the only doctor for more than 100 Ebola patients described his reality as we walked through an Ebola treatment unit in Monrovia, Liberia. Ebola was still spreading fast. Earlier that morning, the makeshift cremation service picked up some of the sixty corpses that had lain for days in sealed body bags, stacked in a large tent that served as a morgue. Three more patients had died overnight. Walking through the unit, I saw a young woman lying face down on a mattress. Her long hair was a tapestry of beautiful, intricately plaited braids, and I thought of how much care she and her family must have taken to create this. I then noticed flies on her, and realized, with horror, that she was one of the three patients who had died the night before. It's an image I can never forget. There weren't enough staff to safely carry the patients who had died to the morgue; other patients lay on thin mattresses on the ground just inches away. More patients were admitted every day, most of them deathly ill. When I returned to the US, I told President Obama that it was like a scene out of Dante. President Obama understood the need for speed. In a speech at the United Nations, he added lines to his prepared remarks, noting that "the slope of the curve . . . is within our control. And if we move fast, even if imperfectly, then that could mean the difference between 10,000, 20,000, 30,000 deaths versus hundreds of thousands or even a million deaths."[7]

In a cringeworthy moment, Dr. Frank Mahoney, then leading our efforts in Liberia, tried to explain the need for fast, flexible funding. President

Obama had arranged a conference call to listen to and encourage staff working on the front lines fighting Ebola. Obama gave brief remarks then invited questions, requests, and suggestions. Mahoney had just met with community leaders in a village where sick and dying Ebola patients had nowhere to go for care. Despite finding a local building that needed only minor repairs, red tape made this impossible. Mahoney was frustrated and he spoke up. And spoke up. And spoke up. Cutting the president off, Mahoney meandered around his point. He explained that what programs often needed was small, simple, but required immediately. Pay to fix a few things to create a makeshift Ebola treatment unit. Pay $100 to rent a hall to train community health workers. Buy gasoline for jeeps or food for trainees' lunch. Mahoney was right: a day, a week, a year, and the opportunity passes. In the Ebola crisis and other epidemics, every minute counts—time is lives. Mahoney saw that speed can make all the difference, and speed requires flexible funding that can be spent immediately.

When Ebola came within days of spreading explosively in Lagos, Nigeria, Mahoney and other CDC staff used flexible funds to create a functional Ebola treatment unit in just ten days, helping stop that outbreak and avert a disaster.[8] This was remarkably fast—such facilities usually take months to establish. When the British military took a leading role in the Ebola response in Sierra Leone, they set up a table with a stack of cash, had workers line up, and, using information the CDC lead doctor provided about who was working and who was not, paid the former and dismissed the latter.

In May 2011, three years before the West Africa Ebola epidemic, an eleven-year-old girl in Luwero, Uganda—less than forty miles from the capital—died after having fever and bleeding. Health workers had suspected Ebola and sent specimens to a Ugandan research institute, which confirmed the case. Because the doctors and nurses caring for the girl isolated her and used protective gear, no one else was infected. The 2014–2016 Ebola epidemic did not have to happen. If Guinea, Sierra Leone, and Liberia had even rudimentary epidemiologists, laboratories, and response capacity, they could have stopped Ebola in months, before it spread to the capital cities and beyond, as Uganda had three years earlier. Digital technologies, artificial intelligence, and advanced laboratory techniques can further accelerate disease detection and response. But speed isn't easy to achieve and maintain, as the US failure to act quickly when COVID struck shows.

LOSING THE RACE AGAINST COVID

The hockey-stick graph (figure 1.1) galvanized US and global action against Ebola in 2014, but in the case of COVID, models were hardly necessary. Explosive spread in China and then in Italy in the last week of February 2020 showed that a deadly pandemic was inevitable.

On Saturday, March 7, 2020, Dr. Deborah Birx, appointed to be the US COVID coordinator the week before, asked me to fly to Washington, DC, to meet with her, Dr. Fauci, two White House officials, and a longtime CDC staffer. The goal was to reset the catastrophically failed US response to COVID. We agreed on banning visits to nursing homes—ground zero for the pandemic and accounting for many avoidable deaths; getting commercial companies focused on testing; and moving toward systematic indoor closures based on real-time data about the virus's spread.

The CDC's lab test had failed, delaying recognition and response to the spread of COVID in the US.[9] Margaret Hoover, President Hoover's great-granddaughter, asked me during an interview on PBS whether the failed CDC lab test cost lives. I mumbled something vague; the honest answer would have been yes, lots of lives. If Seattle and New York City, both hit hard and early and both led by excellent health departments, had been able to test sooner and widely, early spread would have been visible, the cities would likely have closed indoor places much sooner, and disease wouldn't have exploded there and spread so quickly to so many states. Ebola showed that accurate CDC predictions and fast action could prevent a catastrophe; the CDC COVID lab test blunder showed how costly a CDC failure can be.

That same day, March 7, 2020, I met with Dr. Farzad Mostashari. Mostashari had established the phone tracking system that identified the stall in tobacco control progress discussed in chapter 1. He had also helped create the field of syndromic surveillance, a new way to find early signals of outbreaks. Now he was distraught, virtually jumping up and down, showing me data from New York City (figure 6.2).[10] COVID was spreading far

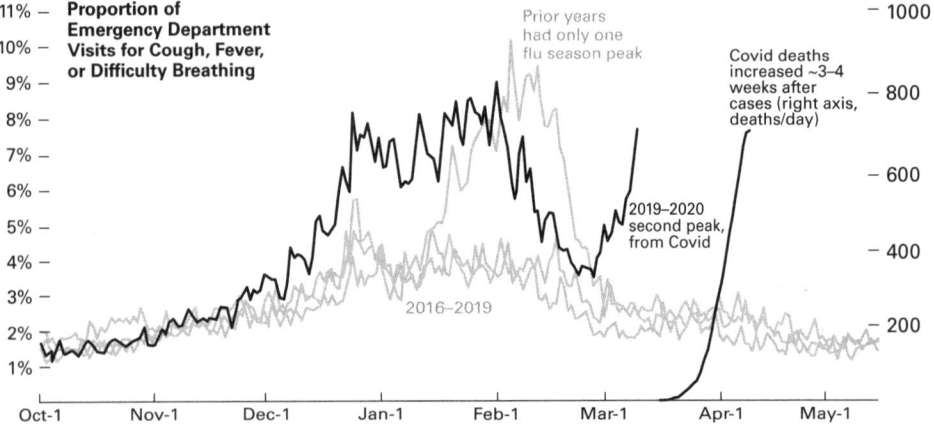

Figure 6.2

The proportion of emergency department visits for respiratory symptoms had one spike in prior years but an unprecedented second spike, from COVID, starting March 2, 2020. Failure of the CDC test kit delayed recognition of and response to spread of the infection. Deaths from COVID rose sharply three to four weeks after rise in respiratory symptoms. Figure created from data made available by the New York City Department of Health and Mental Hygiene.

more widely than anyone realized. Unless the city closed nonessential indoor businesses immediately, tens of thousands of people would die.

Hours later, I sent an email to leadership of my organization, based in New York City, with the subject line: "Telework preparations—IMPORTANT AND TIME SENSITIVE." I'd never sent an email like this before. For the next twelve days, with data showing that COVID was already spreading widely throughout New York City but was invisible because of the lack of accurate tests, we were Cassandras, condemned to foresee future death and destruction but unable to convince others to take action to prevent the catastrophe.

COVID hit both San Francisco and New York City early. Both have superb health departments. In San Francisco, Mayor London Breed listened to her health director and declared a state of emergency before their first case was detected.[11] New York City Mayor Bill de Blasio waited to declare a state of emergency until nearly 100 cases had been reported.[12] Mayor Breed closed indoor businesses when there were 472 known cases.[13] Mayor de Blasio, ignoring the health department's recommendations, didn't call for business closures until more than ten times that number, 5,000, had been detected.[14] In 2020, New York City's death rate was nine times higher than San Francisco's. Every hour of delay killed New Yorkers.

Drs. Oxiris Barbot and Marci Layton are smart, dedicated, hard-working, and straightforward. Dr. Barbot started at the New York City health department as medical director of the school health program and worked her way up from clinician to become the commissioner. Dr. Layton completed her Epidemic Intelligence Service training in New York City and is an epidemiologist's epidemiologist, revered for her insights and effective action on infectious disease outbreaks of the past quarter century, including West Nile virus, anthrax, the 2009 H1N1 influenza pandemic, Ebola, and more.

Both doctors were frantic. The health department had urged Mayor de Blasio to close indoor places, but the head of the public hospitals told the mayor this wasn't necessary. The hospital chief is smart, well-spoken, and deeply experienced running hospitals but knew nothing about pandemics and wasn't willing to listen. "Our ICUs [intensive care units] can handle anything," he told me repeatedly. "Social distancing is unproven. It's not going to work, and we won't be able to run the city." Without test results, the health department couldn't motivate the mayor to act.

Getting political leaders to listen to public health advice is hard, as President Trump and Mayor de Blasio, diametrically opposed on the political spectrum, demonstrated. On March 9, the mayor said, "It's not people . . . at a conference" who are at risk.[15] On the morning of March 12, de Blasio urged Broadway theaters and Madison Square Garden to stay open (the people who ran these places had better sense, announcing closures that afternoon);[16] on March 15, he encouraged New Yorkers to go out to bars;[17] and on March 16, he traveled to and worked out at his favorite gym in Brooklyn.[18]

Exponential growth is a difficult concept to grasp. COVID cases were doubling every two to three days. Day and night, my Brooklyn apartment echoed with the wails of ambulance sirens. COVID killed 23,000 New Yorkers in the first wave—twice as many people as Ebola killed in all of West Africa in the 2014–2016 epidemic.[19] Finally, on March 20, Governor

Cuomo announced closure, starting on March 22.[20] If the delay had been a few days longer, COVID would have killed 50,000 New Yorkers. A week or so longer, 100,000. But a week or ten days less delay would have prevented at least 10,000 deaths.

Hindsight is 20/20, but this wasn't hindsight. Dr. Mostashari, whose tracking system sounded the alarm in early March, urged closure on March 7.[21] Public health practice, like medical practice, isn't just about data; experience matters.[22] An average surgeon who performs hundreds of the same operation has better outcomes than a virtuoso surgeon who performs the operation rarely. The best surgeons operate often, learn from their mistakes, and have an intuitive feel, based on extensive experience, for what to do when faced with a new and dangerous situation. Similarly, the most reliable public health advice is likely to come from an epidemiologist who has spent years responding to outbreaks and has learned from successes and failures. Rational, explicit knowledge is only part of what experience provides; tacit knowledge that informs our perceptions and judgments also matters.[23] This tacit knowledge—another aspect of the art and science of data interpretation discussed in chapter 3—allowed experienced public health experts including Marci Layton and Nancy Messonnier to sense that the COVID pandemic was coming.

While the Trump and DeBlasio administrations fatally delayed action, countries throughout Africa got ahead of the virus. With support from Resolve to Save Lives, they established rapid response funds. Fifteen countries in Africa quickly established their own national incident management system. In just hours, public health leaders could send teams to investigate suspected outbreaks, train nurses in disease investigation and doctors to prevent the spread of infection, buy hand sanitizer, make masks, and limit spread so cases didn't overwhelm their health care system. In an epidemic, a few thousand dollars for a rapid response team today can do more good than few million dollars in a few weeks.[24]

Uganda's COVID response shows what was possible. By July 1, 2020, Uganda had set up screening at its borders that kept out more than 1,100 truck drivers with COVID. Uganda mandated mask-wearing and ensured that use was near universal. It identified and quarantined more than 200 returning travelers with COVID, diagnosed 927 cases, identified more than ten contacts for each case, and tracked nearly every contact. By early July, a hundred days after Uganda's first case, it had fewer total cases than the US had every thirty minutes—a cumulative rate approximately 10,000 times lower than the US rate.

In an epidemic, leaders must always make decisions before perfect information is available. Drs. Barbot and Layton knew what was needed, but Mayor de Blasio's intransigence condemned them to watch the city fail to follow public health advice and then to manage the deaths that followed.

Operation Warp Speed is one standout success in the first Trump administration's management of COVID—it accelerated development of effective vaccines by supporting multiple vaccine approaches. This resulted in vaccines being developed, clinically tested through a standard protocol, and available in record time. Operation Warp Speed shows that with focus, funding, and partnerships, rapid progress is possible.

The global target of 7-1-7 for early outbreak detection, notification, and response accelerates preparedness. It's a simple way to increase accountability and advocacy: Identify every suspected outbreak within 7 days of emergence, report to public health authorities within 1 day, and respond effectively—defined by objective benchmarks—within 7 days.[25] The 7-1-7 target helps break the cycle of endless planning, instead taking a "find a problem, fix a problem" approach, assessing performance in reality rather than on paper.[26] If countries use the target to improve systems after each event, a missed outbreak that grows into an epidemic will be rare.

Simplicity and speed make scale possible. Scale—reaching most or nearly all the people in need—can avert predicted disasters.

SCALE

Many good ideas fail to scale. On a visit in rural Uganda, as I entered a tent, my eyes watered and throat clenched; the heat was oppressive and the soot suffocating. Women were cooking on an open woodstove, as do millions of women in Africa and Asia. Cooking with wood, coal, or dung emits toxic fumes.

More efficient cookstoves pollute less. In a laboratory, these stoves work well. They reduce the amount of fuel needed, so families will save money and effort and want to use them, which will reduce the amount of soot (particulate matter known as PM 2.5) released. There are enormous potential benefits. Less pneumonia.[27] Less deforestation. Less risk of violence when women walk into the forest to gather wood. Less pollution. Fewer house fires. Slower climate change. There's just one problem: In practice, this type of improved cookstove doesn't work. For practical reasons ranging from ease of use to cultural acceptance, this type of stove can't be scaled.

Doctors treat patients one at a time; public health specialists treat entire communities. Advocates and clinicians may maximize benefit for individuals but reach few people. Scalable programs reach entire communities. But scale isn't enough—it's essential to scale programs that are effective. The Burden × Amenability calculation is crucial to prioritize which intervention to scale.

If an intervention has scaled somewhere, it's clearly scalable. In the case of safer cooking, using propane or butane fuel, known as LPG (liquefied petroleum gas) is a scalable replacement for wood, coal, and dung—more than a billion people around the world already cook with it. In Nigeria, more than 85 percent of families cook with soot-producing fuels, and this kills an estimated 100,000 people every year. These fatalities are invisible—they don't appear on any death certificate, and identifying any individual death from cooking fuel is difficult. Replacing wood and other solid fuels with LPG would save lives and reduce climate change.

LPG isn't perfect: It produces small amounts of harmful gases such as carbon monoxide, it requires regulated markets and reasonable costs, and corruption issuing licenses and setting rates must be minimized. It requires changes in cooking habits and cultural expectations. Unfortunately, it replaces one carbon-based fuel with another. Although induction stoves powered by solar energy are even more climate-friendly, they can't be used in most areas that use solid, polluting fuels because the electrical supply isn't reliable. An intervention that can be scaled might not be; economic, practical, and philosophical reasons may prevent LPG scale-up.

Scale often requires strong political leadership. When President George W. Bush launched the President's Emergency Plan for AIDS Relief (PEPFAR)

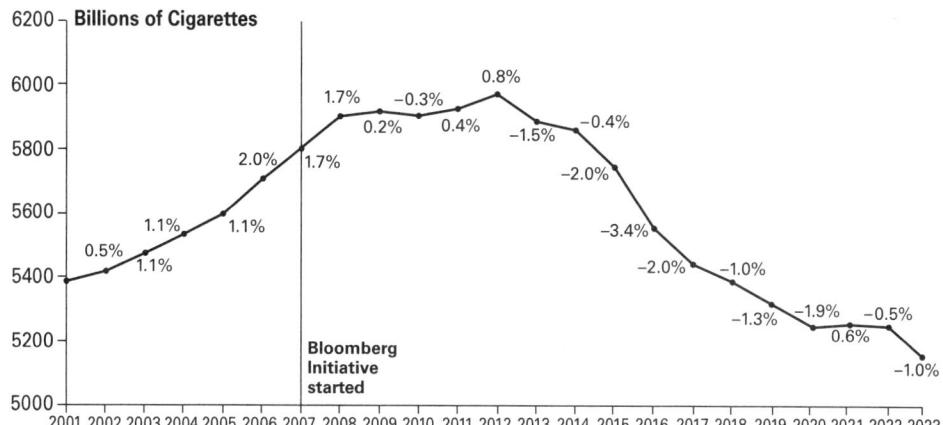

Figure 6.3

Global cigarette sales decline after launch of the Bloomberg Initiative to Reduce Tobacco Use. Despite the steady increase in the number of adults in the world, implementation of the WHO MPOWER strategy in more than 100 countries has led to steady decreases in cigarette sales. Reproduced with permission from Bloomberg Philanthropies.

in 2003, few imagined that by 2025, the program would have prevented 25 million deaths from AIDS. When more than seventy heads of state committed to progress at the 1980 World Summit for Children, they catalyzed progress vaccinating children that has prevented tens of millions of childhood deaths.[28] The Bloomberg Initiative to Reduce Tobacco Use has helped more than one hundred countries implement effective programs, reducing the global smoking rate from 22.7 percent to 17.5 percent; smokers bought 750 billion fewer cigarettes in 2021 than a decade earlier (figure 6.3).[29] The decrease will prevent at least thirty-five million deaths.[30]

Misguided concern about sustainability can be paralyzing and is a common barrier to scaling up health programs. By implementing programs well, success can breed success. Advocates and champions of the program get stronger. Operational habits get established. Political commitment grows. A balanced approach that considers both short-term needs and long-term sustainability can lead to effective and lasting programs. Policy change is a particularly efficient way to sustain progress. Tobacco control programs from the MPOWER technical package (chapter 3) are nearly always irreversible: Once implemented, despite the efforts of tobacco company lobbyists, very few areas reverse smoke-free public places, graphic warning labels on cigarette packs, or advertising bans.

Eradication programs are the ultimate in scale and sustainability: for everyone and forever. Global elimination of artificial trans fat is likely to be irreversible: No child born after global elimination will get exposed to this toxic, artificial, unnecessary chemical. But to succeed, it's essential to get both the technical package and the process of scale-up right.

TIPPING THE SCALES TOWARD SCALABILITY

Success is more likely with strong institutions, a strategic plan, adaptation to the local context, and engaged communities. In addition, simplicity, effective advocacy—including community participation and pressure—and rigorous monitoring to adjust during scale-up increase the odds of success. Recruiting opinion leaders and coalitions of organizations further increases the potential for expansion.[31] The smallpox eradication program demonstrated the importance of adapting as a program grows, innovating to incorporate new technologies and addressing new challenges, opportunities, and political developments.

Successful programs almost always have a support team: "a group of professionals—either inside or outside government, either formally designated or not—who facilitated the scaling-up process."[32] This team can help with advocacy, technical assistance, training, and resource mobilization. Donors fund most such teams. A support team enables countries to achieve the goals they set for themselves, and effective teams build national capacity to sustain progress.

Templates facilitate scale by increasing efficiency and consistency, and by improving evaluation. A template can include examples of protocols, training tools, digital resources, and—perhaps most importantly—standard indicators to monitor and improve the program. Each area or country may adapt and adjust the template to its context. This is the process of scaling, but a process can only succeed if the content can be scaled.

Dr. David Olds, an earnest, kind pediatrician, worked for decades to develop and rigorously study a program to improve the health and social outcomes of children of low-income mothers. Just as Styblo worked for decades to establish the strategy for tuberculosis control, Olds created, optimized, and carefully documented the effectiveness of the Nurse-Family Partnership (NFP).[33]

The NFP trains nurses to support and guide low-income women starting in pregnancy and continuing through the child's second year. Each visit follows a detailed curriculum, with topics for the nurse to discuss and interventions to deliver. Olds proved that the NFP increases about everything you'd want to increase and decreases everything you'd want to decrease. Less child abuse and neglect. Fewer emergency department visits for injuries and poisonings. Better childhood language acquisition. Fewer subsequent unplanned pregnancies. Less crime. Higher maternal employment rates. More economic self-sufficiency.[34] New York City tried to scale up the NFP. Despite our best efforts, the program never scaled to reach more than a small proportion (approximately 10 percent) of the mothers most in need.

David Olds and Karel Styblo each created standardized, rigorously proven technical packages. Styblo's tuberculosis control system, used in more than 150 countries, has improved diagnosis, treatment, and monitoring of more than a hundred million patients. In contrast, Olds's NFP reaches only a small proportion of those in need. Table 6.1 summarizes reasons Styblo's system scaled and Olds's didn't. NFP, although transformational for many families, hasn't yet scaled anywhere. (Other home visitation models may be more scalable.)

Scalability depends on scientific progress, operational excellence, and political courage. The PEPFAR and global immunization programs required scientific advances—better medications and vaccines—and also money: political leaders who match verbal commitments with dollars. Both also required effective management to translate the money and scientific breakthroughs into programs that save lives. In contrast, tobacco control requires primarily political courage. Increased taxes on tobacco raise government revenue; governments must be willing to stand up to powerful tobacco companies.

Many programs that have scaled need to do even more, and other programs are ready to scale but haven't. Tens of thousands of cases of severe birth

Table 6.1

Reasons tuberculosis control, but not the Nurse-Family Partnership, has reached scale

Feature	Tuberculosis control program	Nurse-Family Partnership
Endorsements	The WHO endorsed and promoted, catalyzing global progress	Many organizations endorsed the program, but no authoritative government body unambiguously recommended and promoted it
Simplicity	Simple diagnosis, treatment, and monitoring; implementable by workers with a high school education	Requires nurses; complex and harder to implement
Affordability	Cost-effective and became more affordable (<$30/patient) at scale, with large cost reductions for lab equipment and medications as volumes increased	Although cost-effective, $30,000 or more per mother-child pair with minimal economies of scale; costs and complexity increase with expansion
Addresses a felt need	Serves patients with acute, identifiable needs who seek care	Beneficiaries appreciate the services, but don't feel an acute need
Political salience	Benefits of cured patients are immediate, measurable, and easy to communicate	Benefits are long-term, harder to document and communicate, and less appealing for short-term political horizons

defects could be prevented each year by folic acid fortification of flour, salt, and other foods.[35] Replacement of wood, coal, and dung for cooking with propane canisters or electric stoves could reduce deforestation, slow global warming, and prevent pneumonia and heart disease for millions of people.[36] Further improvements in water and sanitation could increase child survival and hasten economic progress.[37] Increased tobacco taxes could prevent tens of millions of people from dying young. Low-cost, safe treatment of hypertension could prevent five million heart attacks and strokes each year.[38]

TRIAD: SIMPLICITY, SPEED, AND SCALE

Simplicity, speed, and scale were all necessary to stop the 2014–2016 Ebola epidemic. On my first visit to West Africa during the epidemic, I traveled deep into hot, humid villages where CDC Epidemic Intelligence Service officers worked around the clock. Hospitals couldn't keep up with the increasing number of patients unless we stopped the virus from spreading. The program had to find cases sooner, isolate them, quarantine their contacts, and ensure safe burial. But after reviewing the officers' work, I was appalled. They had spent weeks frantically entering data from multipage intake forms of patients with suspected or confirmed Ebola. They were working around the clock and as quickly as they could, but no one had checked or analyzed the data. No one had assessed whether all the information was required. I ordered staff to simplify and create a one-page intake form immediately, with only essential information . . . but it took more than a month to develop the revised form. Since we failed to simplify and adjust quickly to the exponential increase in case numbers, the outbreak expanded faster than our response. We were failing.

Then, working with doctors, community leaders, and global partners, the team developed a plan: Get the corpses—teeming with Ebola—out of houses and off the streets and provide safe and dignified burial services. Isolate and assess sick patients quickly; if they had Ebola, isolate them anywhere—hospitals, community centers, and, when possible, Ebola treatment units. Once the explosive spread stopped, expand classic public health measures used for tuberculosis and smallpox: Find and isolate patients quickly, track their contacts, and stop spread in health care facilities.

Two superb CDC epidemiologists, Drs. Frank Mahoney and Kim Lindblade, alongside CDC and Liberian colleagues, established the plan: Rapid Isolation and Treatment of Ebola (RITE). They learned that if they sent a team within a day or two of a new case or cluster of Ebola, they could stop spread within weeks instead of months, limiting cases to a handful rather than hundreds. This approach was particularly important for rural communities, which are often neglected. Dr. Lindblade summarized the approach: "Every detail is important." With RITE, communities stopped outbreaks twice as fast—twenty-five instead of fifty-three days—and nearly tripled patient survival, from 28 percent to 81 percent.[39]

Ebola had erupted in societies emerging from war and dictatorship. Most adults were not literate and had deep distrust of government and of modern medicine. Patient by patient, contact by contact, cluster by cluster, the core public health approach worked. Hans Rosling, who worked in Liberia to support the response to Ebola, recognized the fundamental importance of outreach workers and government staff:

The fight against the lethal Ebola virus was won not by an individual heroic leader, or even by one heroic organization like Médecins Sans Frontières or UNICEF. It was won prosaically and undramatically by government staff and local health workers who created public health campaigns that changed ancient funeral practices in a matter of days; risked their lives to treat dying patients; and did the cumbersome, dangerous, and delicate work of finding and isolating all the people who had been in contact with them. Brave and patient servants of a functioning society, rarely ever mentioned—but the true saviors of the world.[40]

Public health staff in all three countries persisted until they stopped the epidemic in every community.

Simplicity, speed, and scale stopped the Ebola epidemic and are necessary for the create phase of the See/Believe/Create formula to save the most lives. But even a simple, well-managed program will fail unless it communicates effectively. Every part of the formula requires effective communication—to convince others of what they're seeing, spread the belief that change is possible, and implement programs that overcome the odds against successful public health action.

7 COMMUNICATION

A word after a word after a word is power.
—Margaret Atwood

As I drove up the long, dusty dirt driveway toward a ramshackle house in Douglas, Tennessee, it dawned on me, gradually, that what the young girl on the porch was pointing at me was a shotgun. She was alone in the house and scared. A group in Nashville had sent me, just out of college in my first public health job, to solve a mystery: People in Douglas were poor and sick, but the new health clinic was empty. Why were so few people using the clinic?

Douglas was an unusual community in some ways and all too normal in others. Eleanor Roosevelt took an interest in the area and championed New Deal farming programs. At that time, seventy years after the end of the Civil War, many people were still sharecropping. A farmer showed me where he had torn down an old tool shack. He didn't know how good the soil would be, so he added fertilizer; his corn grew more than twenty feet high, so far over his head that he had to chop down the stalks to harvest it. The rolling hills and rich, fertile soil contrasted with the poverty of the area. Generations after Black farmers became landowners, the area remained poor, progress derailed by subdivided plots, hostility of White farmers and institutions, and agricultural consolidation. Some houses lacked electricity and indoor plumbing. I had never seen such destitution in the United States—the term *tar shack* doesn't capture the reality. Walls and ceilings made of mud, sticks, and sheets of tar paper that were rough to touch and gave off a pungent chemical smell in the summer heat. Dirt floors that were uneven and often damp. Health problems ranging from skin infections to painful arthritis to cancer went undiagnosed and untreated. In jarring contrast, the gleaming new clinic stood largely empty.

The community health clinic movement, part of the Great Society efforts of the 1960s and 1970s, encouraged communities to organize and request a clinic. Douglas had done so—over the objections of White physicians from the nearby town, who feared competition. In addition to an ice cream factory and a famous ribs restaurant, the area now had its health clinic. We had to solve the mystery of why so few people used it.

With census maps, we identified every house served by the clinic and selected a random sample of households to interview. Researchers rarely use random sampling for household surveys—it's too labor-intensive and there are more efficient ways to get representative data—but at the time I didn't know any better. The house-to-house survey of 374 families (with just one shotgun refusal) solved the mystery. Even in this community of 14,080 people where everyone supposedly knew everything going on, half didn't know the clinic existed, four out of five didn't know a visit could cost only $10, and almost no one knew the clinic would provide free transportation to and from visits. What's more, the people who *did* know were better off and less likely to need care at the clinic. Poverty isn't just about money—it's also about access to information. The Douglas clinic failed to protect people in the community because it failed to communicate.

Communication can determine whether a life-saving program succeeds or fails. To help people see problems, believe in solutions, and create a healthier future, it's essential to listen carefully and convey messages effectively. Cassandra's inability to convince others of impending tragedy—a communication failure—was the essence of her curse.[1] She warned of impending disasters, but no one saw the future she perceived or believed her predictions. Effective communication is important for warnings, motivation, advocacy, health campaigns, and emergency messages; it starts with getting the message right.

THE RIGHT MESSAGE

The frightening projection of the potential explosion of Ebola cases in West Africa (figure 1.1) helped US and global leaders see the impending disaster. Personal stories—too rarely used to explain public health concepts and recommendations—can also make visible what would otherwise be ignored. Ryan White, a teenager who became a national symbol for HIV/AIDS in the United States, made stigma and the pain it caused more visible—the See part of the formula—and, by doing so, helped reduce this stigma.

Many health risks remain hidden from public awareness until effective communication exposes them. Even after the link had been proven, the severe harms of smoking—including cancer, heart attacks, and lung disease—didn't become apparent until people saw images of diseased organs and heard personal stories of those affected. Similarly, few understood the risks associated with secondhand smoke until graphic ads showed the impact on children, spouses, and others. The tobacco industry hid its deceptive practices until lawsuits and investigative journalism uncovered its lies about the health risks of smoking and the addictiveness of nicotine. With the impending epidemic of Ebola in West Africa, the pain of discrimination against people living with HIV, and the hidden harms, addictiveness, and devious tactics of the tobacco industry, effective communication helped people see what had been invisible.

Words matter. Slight differences in phrasing can lead to large differences in the effectiveness of a message.[2] Frank Luntz, a communications professional, advised the CDC on messaging. His focus groups found *protect* a much more powerful word than *prevent*, were impressed that the CDC works 24/7, and understood avoiding *threats* better than avoiding diseases, conditions, or illnesses. Based on this, Luntz advised us to summarize CDC's mission: "The CDC works 24/7 to protect Americans from threats." It's simple, accurate, easy to understand, and crosses many divides that might otherwise splinter support.

Effective communication is also essential for people to believe progress is possible. Skin cancer seemed to be an inevitable consequence of living in a sunny climate. Then, in 1981, Australia launched a clear, simple

"Slip-Slop-Slap" campaign—"Slip on a shirt, slop on sunscreen, slap on a hat." The campaign showed that everyone had the power to protect themselves. Slip-Slop-Slap changed what people believed was possible, and use of sunscreen and protective clothing increased, leading to a decrease in skin cancer.[3]

Communication can frame the intervention that creates a healthier future. When the New York City health department banned artificial trans fat from restaurants, we didn't call it partially hydrogenated vegetable oil but rather—accurately—an artificial, toxic chemical that can kill you. With that framing, not even the food industry opposed making food trans-fat-free. (And making food trans-fat-free or protecting workers from tobacco smoke sounds better than banning ingredients or making smoking illegal.) Finding the right message requires creativity, inspiration, and also scientific rigor.

If the findings of a study or a recommendation can't be summarized in a headline, either the analysis or the message needs to be improved. A single overriding communication objective (SOCO) can help. A SOCO is a memorable, accurate, strategic one-line summary. For example, "Second-hand smoke kills" or "Don't drink and drive." A health SOCO should not be a glib one-liner that promises the impossible but a clear, accurate message backed by rigorous data. COVID showed that getting the message right can be a matter of life and death.

A FAILURE TO COMMUNICATE

Jacinda Ardern and Donald Trump both led their countries through the first year of the COVID pandemic. Their approaches differed in many ways, but communication was the most important determinant of how many people died. Ardern's approach as prime minister of New Zealand exemplifies how to get the message right so people see an invisible but impending problem, believe they can address it, and do the right thing; Trump's communications undermined all three elements of the See/Believe/Create formula, contributing to hundreds of thousands of preventable deaths. Of the many disastrous aspects of the US response to COVID under the first Trump administration, failure to communicate effectively was likely the costliest in lives lost and economic harm.

Ardern's clear, empathetic, and consistent communication helped people grasp the magnitude of the threat. From the outset, she conveyed the gravity of the pandemic, stating, "We are fortunate to still be some way behind the majority of overseas countries in terms of cases, but the trajectory is clear: act now, or risk the virus taking hold as it has elsewhere."[4] This transparency helped New Zealanders understand the urgency of the situation and the necessary measures to combat it. In contrast, Trump downplayed the virus and assured the public it would "disappear . . . like a miracle."[5] This led to a delayed and disjointed response, with many Americans not grasping the severity of the pandemic until too late.

Ardern also helped instill the belief that the country could address COVID. She communicated a clear plan of action, emphasizing unity and collective responsibility: "We will get through this together, but only if we stick together, so please be strong and be kind."[6] Trump vacillated between irrational reassurance and irresponsible defeatism. After claiming the virus would miraculously disappear, he suggested that it should be allowed to "wash over" the country.[7] These conflicting messages created confusion and fear, undermined confidence in the government's response, and reduced willingness to take protective actions.

When it came to doing the right thing to create a healthier future, Ardern provided clear, evidence-based guidance and modeled the masking and vaccination behaviors she asked of citizens: "This isn't a decision we took lightly, but we know masks protect you and the people around you."[8] She also communicated transparently about vaccine distribution, saying, "Throughout the roll out of the vaccine program, our approach has been to match our vaccination rate with available supply."[9] Her consistent and empathetic communication helped build trust and increase compliance. In contrast, Trump's approach was erratic and often contradicted proven approaches. Despite evidence supporting mask use, Trump publicly downplayed their importance, saying, "I just don't want to wear one myself."[10] His promotion of unproven treatments, including hydroxychloroquine, further eroded trust and contributed to underuse of effective treatments such as Paxlovid. His politicization of the vaccine approval process and lack of a coherent vaccination plan contributed to skepticism, reluctance to be vaccinated, and low vaccine coverage.

New Zealand's COVID mortality rate per population was nearly five times lower than that of the United States. Although weaker primary health care, a less cohesive society, and more chronic illness contributed to the higher rate in the United States, and although protecting an island country is easier, ineffective communication greatly compounded US vulnerabilities. If the United States had managed the pandemic with the same effectiveness as New Zealand, many Americans killed by the virus would still be alive.[11] Any country that fails to organize and communicate effectively risks avoidable deaths and economic devastation from the next pandemic.

Good communication defines an issue, builds trust, and creates ongoing feedback loops so those in power can learn from the public and promote healthy behavior. For decades before the COVID pandemic, leaders in the United States and globally had used CDC's guidelines for communication in a health emergency.[12] These guidelines call for empathy, competence, and honesty; warn against overly reassuring statements; advise giving people useful things to do; and emphasize getting people to work together. The basic concepts are: Be first, be right, be credible. Because knowledge will inevitably increase and recommendations may change, start statements with "Based on what we know now." During the US response to COVID under President Trump, these principles were not just ignored—they were contradicted. Table 7.1 lists the principles of communication in a health emergency and contrasts them with what President Trump actually said.

As early as February 25, 2020, Dr. Nancy Messonnier, CDC's lead scientist for respiratory infections, personalized her concern:

> I had a conversation with my family over breakfast this morning and I told my children that while I didn't think that they were at risk right now, we as a family need to be preparing for significant disruption of our lives.[13]

Then, Cassandra-like, she warned, "Disruption to everyday life may be severe." Her message contradicted the administration's denial, and the Trump administration prohibited her from speaking to the public about the pandemic for the remainder of Trump's first term in office.[14]

Table 7.1

Violations of basic principles of health communication, Trump administration, 2020

Principle	CDC guidance*	Violation in the Trump administration
Be first	"Crises are time-sensitive. Communicating information quickly is crucial. For members of the public, the first source of information often becomes the preferred source."	The Trump administration silenced the CDC after public health officials tried to warn the public about the coming pandemic. Trump claimed, falsely, on February 29, 2020: "We've taken the most aggressive actions to confront the coronavirus. They are the most aggressive taken by any country." The administration delayed for six weeks after the WHO declaration to declare a national emergency, and repeatedly delayed release of CDC guidance.**
Be right	"Accuracy establishes credibility. Information can include what is known, what is not known, and what is being done to fill in the gaps."	President Trump on February 23: "We have it very much under control in this country."
Be credible	"Honesty and truthfulness should not be compromised during crises. Don't over-reassure. Acknowledge uncertainty."	President Trump on February 10: "Looks like by April, you know, in theory, when it gets a little warmer, it miraculously goes away." On February 27: "It's going to disappear. One day, it's like a miracle, it will disappear." On April 23: "I see the disinfectant where it knocks it out in a minute—one minute—and is there a way we can do something like that by injection inside, or almost a cleaning?"
Express empathy	"Crises create harm, and the suffering should be acknowledged in words. Addressing what people are feeling, and the challenges they face, builds trust and rapport. Acknowledge people's fear."	President Trump on March 10: "We're prepared, and we're doing a great job with it. And it will go away. Just stay calm. It will go away." When asked, "What do you say to Americans who are watching you right now who are scared?" Trump replied, "I say that you're a terrible reporter—that's what I say."
Promote action	"Giving people meaningful things to do calms anxiety, helps restore order, and promotes some sense of control."	Despite evidence supporting the use of masks, on April 3, President Trump said, "I just don't want to wear one myself. . . . I'm feeling good. . . . Somehow, I don't see it for myself. I just—I just don't." On April 5: "I would wear one," but only "if I thought it was important." On June 19: "I let people make up their own decision."
Show respect	"Respectful communication is particularly important when people feel vulnerable. Respectful communication promotes cooperation and rapport."	On April 12, President Trump: "When somebody is president of the United States, the authority is total. The governors know that."

*US Department of Health and Human Services and US Centers for Disease Control and Prevention, *Crisis Emergency Risk Communication*.
**Union of Concerned Scientists, "Trump Administration Interfered with CDC's Public Outreach on COVID-19," March 17, 2022, https://www.ucsusa.org/resources/attacks-on-science/trump-administration-interfered-cdcs-public-outreach-covid-19.

It would be hard—perhaps impossible—to violate the CDC principles more completely than President Trump did. The result of Trump's undermining trust in CDC and in science was resistance to sensible control measures, avoidable disease and death, economic setbacks, and decreased confidence in life-saving vaccinations. Poor communication can cost lives.

The Biden administration greatly improved the response to the COVID pandemic, including with a structured incident management system. However, in an effort to ensure messaging consistency, it insisted that CDC doctors be part of White House communications. This eroded trust in the CDC—and reduced vaccination rates—among people who voted against President Biden.[15] This illustrates that it's not only essential to have the right message; having the right messengers—in this case, doctors insulated from entities seen as partisan—is also essential.

THE RIGHT MESSENGER

The right messenger can make all the difference. Jorge, a forty-two-year-old man with hemophilia, had been coughing for months. He entered the downtown Brooklyn tuberculosis clinic, swinging into my examination room on crutches. Tests showed that he had tuberculosis and that it was resistant to the most effective medication. He was from Ecuador, didn't have legal immigration status, worked in an off-the-books factory, and didn't trust our clinic. The best anti-tuberculosis treatment at the time was thrice-weekly medication for nine months. This would have to be given by the clinic's outreach worker, Christian Nwigwe. Nwigwe had been a salesman in Nigeria and was one of the hundreds of outreach workers we employed once we broke the hiring logjam described in chapter 5.

Jorge spoke no English. Despite my passable Spanish, I failed to convince him to meet Nwigwe three times a week. Then Nwigwe, who spoke no Spanish, convinced him. Astonishingly, although they lacked a common language, Nwigwe, conveying deep caring and using the persuasive presence of a salesman, created the trust essential for effective outreach. Every Monday, Wednesday, and Friday at lunchtime, Jorge left his factory and walked, swinging on his crutches, two blocks away, gingerly opening the passenger door of Nwigwe's boxy blue city-issued car. Nwigwe would bring him a sandwich and juice, and Jorge would take his medicines, then walk back to his factory on his crutches. After nine months, we confirmed that Jorge was cured. Nwigwe was the right messenger for Jorge; Terrie Hall was the right messenger for millions of smokers.

Hall was a cheerleader in her North Carolina high school; she also worked on a tobacco farm and began a two-pack-a-day smoking habit. At age forty, she developed oral and throat cancer and began grueling radiation treatments and chemotherapy. Hall, who was fierce and funny, volunteered to tell her story when CDC launched the Tips from Former Smokers campaign. The day before she died, at age fifty-three, she insisted that we film her—determined to help others avoid the suffering she had experienced. Real-life stories show the disability and disfigurement smoking causes and help smokers quit. (Showing either death or the health benefits of quitting don't motivate change as effectively.) Hall's powerful message helped tens of thousands of smokers quit and saved many more lives than most doctors will save in their entire career.[16]

Different messengers are right for different communities. During the West Africa Ebola epidemic of 2014–2016, steady progress became possible only when response teams understood community perceptions and enlisted community leaders to speak with patients and families to encourage medical treatment and safe and dignified burial.[17] Black patients in the United States have better health outcomes when treated by Black doctors.[18] Similarly, community health workers from within the population they serve can improve vaccination rates and management of hypertension and other conditions.

THE RIGHT AUDIENCE

Finding the right audience is also essential to the effective communication component of creating a healthier future. To ban trans fats in New York City, we first tried educating the public. This failed. It just wasn't possible to get people riled up about something they hadn't heard of, didn't know was in their food, and couldn't see, taste, or feel. We got the regulation passed when we shifted our strategy and targeted decision-makers in City Hall and the Board of Health, providing technical data that proved that banning trans fat would save lives without harming the economy. And by communicating effectively with restaurant operators and suppliers—including listening carefully to their valid concerns—we smoothed implementation of the regulation.[19] This experience informed the global approach that has helped dozens of countries ban trans fat: Focus on decision-makers rather than try, against all odds, to generate a groundswell of public opinion to ban something most people have never heard of.

Identifying the right audience and tailoring communication to different communities is essential to change perceptions, influence behaviors, and improve health outcomes. But the right message and messenger aren't static. Effective communication requires feedback loops to refine messages and understand changing perceptions and concerns. This means collecting data and adjusting so communication strategies remain effective. Listening, as we did to the people in Douglas, Tennessee, often reveals surprising and essential information.

During the COVID pandemic, Resolve to Save Lives created the Partnership for Evidence-Based Response to COVID. Over several years, the Partnership conducted four large phone surveys and collected data from other sources across nineteen countries in Africa.[20] The data helped governments hone their responses by providing real-time insights into public perceptions and behaviors, allowing them to increase the effectiveness of messages about preventive measures, vaccines, and other public health guidance. For example, the surveys identified severe economic hardship from closures of open-air markets; quick action to keep these markets functioning increased receptivity to reasonable and realistic recommendations for preventive behaviors.

Effective communication includes "earned" media—news articles. Quick, credible, and effective messages can frame an issue. Most reporters are interested in learning and want to produce accurate stories. Speaking with media and the public with clear, accurate, engaging information requires in-depth understanding of an issue and the ability to explain it simply. Advocates transformed the public perception of drunk driving from inevitable or humorous to irresponsible behavior that killed children; this triggered life-saving laws and cultural shifts such as designated drivers. When accused of trying to ban guns, gun safety advocates note that cars were not banned but became safer because of regulation and design improvements, and that analogous improvements could reduce injuries and deaths from guns. Simple and clear framing can make progress possible. If the staff of the Douglas clinic had conveyed that it was there, affordable, and provided free transportation, they could have prevented more illnesses and deaths.

Social media is a rapidly changing frontier. New voices able to summarize complex science accurately and crisply have emerged—as have irresponsible people who oversimplify and sensationalize. Public health can partner with responsible social media influencers to reach multiple audiences and better address the deadly challenge of misinformation.

MISINFORMATION

In minutes, misinformation can reach millions of people and reverse years of public health communication. Nearly 200 years ago, Ben Franklin confronted this challenge when his four-year-old child died; there were rumors that smallpox vaccination had killed the boy. Franklin published a statement in his newspaper trying to block the spread of misinformation, explaining that his child died from smallpox and that the child had not received the inoculation.[21]

Misinformation about vaccines is as old as vaccines themselves, but social media accelerates the spread of anti-vaccination and other rumors, and artificial intelligence can make the spread much worse. As vaccines succeed, cases decline, and as cases decline, parental willingness to vaccinate their children also declines—another deadly manifestation of the invisibility of risk and of progress. For any one child, not being vaccinated would be safer than being vaccinated—but only if all other parents have their children vaccinated. Vaccination therefore presents the classic free-rider dilemma, a collective action problem.[22] Virtually every vaccination campaign has faced resistance, rumor, and rejection. In the 1860s, mobs in Massachusetts and Virginia burned down the houses of doctors who provided smallpox inoculation.[23]

Franklin became a strong advocate for vaccination. He knew that the most effective approach would be to help others imagine the horror of having failed to vaccinate a child and then feeling responsible for their child's death. People can break their personal Cassandra curse when they see a horrific but preventable future. Nearly half a century after his son's death, in the hope of encouraging parents to vaccinate their children, Franklin wrote in his autobiography:

> In 1736 I lost one of my Sons, a fine Boy of 4 Years old, taken by the Small Pox in the common way. I long regretted that I had not given it to him by Inoculation, which I mention for the Sake of Parents, who omit that Operation on the Supposition that they should never forgive themselves if a Child died under it; my Example showing that the Regret may be the same either way, and that therefore the safer should be chosen.[24]

Preventing the harms of misinformation is hard. We must expose the profit motives of individuals and companies that spread it and hold social media companies accountable, including through greater transparency about their algorithms. Prevention works better than correction: Establishing trusted communication channels before an emergency is more effective than only playing whack-a-mole with rumors. Stronger defenses require long-term investments in education to promote critical thinking, investigative journalism, and reliable information sources. It will also help to acknowledge mistakes when we make them, admit what we don't know, listen sincerely, and speak clearly. But building trust may be the most powerful antidote to misinformation.

TRUST

Do Americans trust the government to do what is right all or most of the time? For more than sixty-five years, the Pew Research Center has asked this question. From a high of nearly 80 percent in the early 1960s, the proportion fell steadily, increasing only during the prosperous Clinton years and immediately after the 9/11 attacks. During Trump's first presidency, the level dropped to record lows—17 percent—and, for the first time, to single digits among Black Americans.[25] It has stayed below 20 percent. Trust is vital to stop infectious diseases, but it's the one thing that can't be surged into a community during an emergency. With a trustworthy message conveyed by a trusted messenger to the right audience, people are much more likely to follow recommendations to change behavior, seek care, and accept treatment—or vaccination.[26]

Trust is indispensable for vaccine acceptance. Vaccines, along with clean water and sanitation, are among humanity's greatest discoveries. They have saved hundreds of millions of lives, prevented massive suffering and disability, and facilitated economic progress in every part of the world. Like any invention, vaccines aren't perfect. Injections can hurt and, rarely, cause severe adverse reactions. They don't protect everyone. Some must be given multiple times to be effective. A global resurgence of measles occurred partly because of misinformation spread by the fraudulent, disproven claim that measles vaccination causes autism.[27] Without stronger trust in vaccines, killer diseases including measles, diphtheria, rotavirus, and pneumonia could again kill and disable millions of children.

Economist John Maynard Keynes reputedly said, "When the facts change, I change my mind. What do you do, sir?" If good communication fails to prepare people for changes as health crises evolve, the answer to that question may be "Stop believing public health officials." Maintaining trust requires explicit recognition of both our desire for certainty and the inevitability that new information will change our understanding.

At the outset of the COVID pandemic, government leaders lost trust when they did not state one of the main reasons they didn't recommend masks for the public: There weren't enough for health care workers. This simply wasn't honest. The recommendation changed when it became clear that half or more of infections are spread before people have symptoms, that masks can substantially reduce spread, and when there were more masks available. Poor communication, lack of understanding of how science works, and partisan politics led to confusion, controversy, and avoidable spread of COVID. In East Asian countries including Japan and South Korea, mask-wearing has long been common and socially accepted; this likely accounts for much of the fivefold lower death rate from COVID in those countries. In the United States, mask-wearing became politicized, with irrational mandates to wear masks outdoors and failure to communicate that masks could facilitate the faster and safer reopening of most businesses.

Public health agencies made mistakes during the pandemic, ranging from the CDC lab test error to muddled messages on masks, but the biggest mistake was political leaders' failure to follow public health guidance. In countries where public health leaders, supported by political leaders, based their recommendations on the latest available data, there were fewer deaths, fewer job losses, and less economic devastation.[28]

Many people in Black communities distrust health programs. This is in part the legacy of the inexcusable Tuskegee experiment, during which public health doctors and nurses monitored Black men with untreated syphilis from 1932 to 1972 as they got sicker and failed to provide a cure when one became available. Public health experts now generally understand the importance of sensitive outreach to Black communities. But many of the same experts have been slow to recognize that other communities are also deeply alienated from public health and disinclined to believe predictions of illness or to follow recommendations. In focus groups, Americans reluctant to get vaccinated against COVID expressed anger and deep frustration. They felt unheard and disrespected: No one had addressed, much less answered, their legitimate questions.[29] To build trust, communication must reach every community—listening to concerns, answering questions, and providing tailored messages and messengers.

Trust can be lost in an instant but restored only slowly. Timely, accurate, useful communication with the right messengers and messages is essential. Openness about whether programs are succeeding or failing is necessary. Listening—understanding, empathizing, and addressing concerns—is important. But communication alone, no matter how effective, won't restore trust. Public health must solve—and be seen to solve—problems the public believes are important.

After making a problem and its solution visible and convincing people it's fixable (chapters 1–4), successful programs manage well through effective organization, with simplicity, speed, and scale (chapters 5 and 6). Effective communication, described in this chapter, accelerates and facilitates progress. But fundamentally, public health decisions are political decisions. Unless public health gains political power, it can't implement the formula and won't save lives.

8 PROGRESS DESPITE OPPOSITION

Mark Twain wrote, "Thunder is good, thunder is impressive, but it's lightning that does the work."

In public health, it's law and regulation that do the work.
—Mayor Michael Bloomberg

Smoke-free restaurants and bars. Steep increases in tobacco taxes. Trans fats banned. All good progress, but we were losing the battle against obesity. Soda was a clear culprit. As fruits and vegetables became more expensive, soda got cheaper. Americans hadn't decreased their physical activity much but were consuming 300 kilocalories more per day, and soda accounted for about half of that increase. A tax would reduce consumption and seemed like a no-brainer: protect children, combat rising rates of obesity and diabetes, reduce health care costs, and raise revenue.

In April 2009, a colleague and I published an article in the *New England Journal of Medicine* titled "Ounces of Prevention," making the case for a penny-an-ounce tax on soda.[1] Soon after I joined the Obama administration, the president and his budget director mused about taxing soda nationally.[2] Working with community groups and university scientists, we supported a New York State initiative to levy a one cent per ounce tax on sugar-sweetened beverages. In 2010, Governor David Patterson announced the proposal, and Mayor Bloomberg supported it strongly.

Then reality fought back, hard. The soda industry's front group, the American Beverage Association, launched an assault on the proposal: They said the tax would be a regressive burden on consumers and a threat to jobs, small businesses, and the economy. They lobbied, advertised, donated money to politicians, and funded "astroturf" groups that pretended to be grassroots organizations. Albany killed the legislation and the Obama administration dropped the idea.

Soda taxes save lives, reduce health care costs, and generate government revenue. But it's almost impossible to get a soda tax approved. Why? Opposition.

WINNERS AND LOSERS

Policies create winners and losers. Coca-Cola, PepsiCo, and other powerful companies would lose big from a soda tax. Taxes reduce consumption of soda and cut into sales and profits. There are many more winners: families that don't have to deal with obesity, health care systems with lower costs, and businesses that become more productive when their workers are less likely to be disabled. But the winners won't know about the benefits, most of which are far in the future. And, unlike Coke and Pepsi, the winners aren't well organized and don't have much influence on the politicians who decide whether or not to approve the tax. Mike Bloomberg understands this dynamic well; when I commented that his global public health philanthropy had saved 35 million lives, he grinned and quipped, "Yeah, but not one of those people ever thanked me."

This is an example of the challenge of concentrated losses and diffuse benefits, and, as discussed in chapter 2, it results from the prevention paradox: The biggest health improvements come from small changes across entire populations. Counteracting concentrated opposition is essential to the *Create* part of the formula to save the most lives. This is hard, but it's not impossible.

If the winners from public health policy organize, they can prevail. That's how New York City got clean water, starting in the 1840s after cholera epidemics killed thousands and led as many as a third of residents to flee the city. Businesses struggled with unreliable and contaminated water supplies, and water shortage led to a devastating fire. Upstate farmers blocked reservoir construction to protect their land—they were the concentrated losers from a policy that would benefit large numbers of people. Then, an alliance of merchants, bankers, public health advocates, and newspaper editors organized; they feared that New York City would lose its preeminence as a commercial center. New York City leaders created a great reservoir system that gave the city pristine water, saved lives, and promoted growth. To do so, they seized the farmers' land and paid paltry compensation.[3]

Losers from actions that protect health are often much more powerful than those upstate farmers: companies that sell tobacco, alcohol, and unhealthy food; hospitals that have to spend more on infection prevention or disease reporting; agribusinesses that have to change what or how they produce.

During Mayor Bloomberg's first term, we increased the tobacco tax, made restaurants, bars, and other public places smoke-free, opened new syringe exchange programs, and more. These had been big fights, and, although all were effective and increasingly popular—or at least accepted—Bloomberg remembered the "one-fingered waves" he received from voters who wanted to smoke in bars. The politics of public health is brutal. When Mayor Bloomberg ran for reelection in 2005, I asked Shea Fink, his blunt, often profane, and always-fun-to-work-with scheduler, what I could do to help. "Oh," Fink said, "here's what you can do to help. Let us put duct tape over your mouth and lock you in a closet until after the election." After Bloomberg won, he called all commissioners into the ornate "Blue Room" at City Hall and told us that in the second term we needed to do more unpopular things. His 72 percent approval rating, he continued, indicated that we weren't making the kind of hard choices that he—having self-financed his election—was uniquely positioned to make. If we did what we were supposed to do, his popularity rating should decrease. From the back of the room, Ed Skyler, the mayor's brash communications director, shouted: "We're counting on you, Tom!"

To create a healthy future, understanding who wins and who loses is important, but that's not the same as understanding how to make change happen. After all, Coke and Pepsi don't pass laws—only politicians can do that. Sometimes politicians will support public health. That requires figuring out who makes the decisions, when, and how to influence them.

In 1998, despite government backing, support from the World Bank, and Karel Styblo's proven strategy, India's new tuberculosis control program was in deep trouble. Stopping a program is much easier than starting one—many people and institutions can block progress. The World Bank insisted that the government buy medications more transparently. This threatened powerful interests—drug companies with an inside track on large contracts, along with the staff, consultants, and others who benefited from these contracts. The losers from better procurement—powerful drug companies—blocked change. The winners—tuberculosis patients who would receive treatment—were unaware of the struggle, not organized, and powerless. Most hadn't even developed tuberculosis yet! Patients on treatment would soon run out of medicines. It would only be possible to overcome the powerful drug companies by getting to those who could make the decision.

DECIDERS AND INFLUENCERS

It was 10:00 p.m. in New Delhi, India, and I was crouching out of sight on the floorboards of a creaky Ambassador car across the street from a politician close to then-Prime Minister Atal Vajpayee. In the car: a laptop and portable printer, in case the politician asked for revisions to the question-and-answer sheet we had drafted. The politician could influence the prime minister, who in turn could respond to a question in parliament the next morning. Dr. Khatri, my Indian counterpart, had sheepishly asked me to crouch down; seeing me could tip off companies opposed to the procurement reform that would restart the program. The strategy worked. The next day, in response to the question, the prime minister made a statement in parliament that got the program back on track.

Khatri knew that this politician could influence the prime minister. Khatri also knew that a statement in parliament would force those blocking the program to relent. Every effort to improve health programs or policies must confront or enlist people who make decisions and those who influence them. Progress requires identifying, reaching, and recruiting deciders and influencers. That, in turn, requires understanding the landscape—what the process is, who can influence and make decisions and when, what the constraints are, and what effects elections, budgets, economic changes, personal connections, media, social movements, and other factors have on the possibilities.

At a critical moment in the fight against smallpox in India in the 1970s, there were thousands of outbreaks. Bill Foege requested approval to expand the team of international epidemiologists by bringing in another fifty, hoping the government would approve ten. Foege sensed that the health minister didn't like him and asked his Indian counterpart why. Foege and the program director had a good enough relationship for his counterpart to be frank: "The minister says we don't need any foreigners to tell us about smallpox. We have many experts who have more experience, so why do we need them? And besides, they come from places that don't even have smallpox!" Foege replied: "The minister is absolutely correct. You do have more experience and more experts. But you might ask the minister one question: Does he want smallpox eradicated on his watch or on his successor's?"

Asked this question, the minister approved fifty more international epidemiologists—and required that each be paired with and train an Indian epidemiologist. Foege had hoped to have ten additional highly qualified staff and now he had one hundred. This made it possible to track and stop thousands of outbreaks that would otherwise have delayed the victory over smallpox in India for months, if not years. Progress requires getting to the right person, in the right way, at the right time—and not just to stop infectious diseases such as smallpox.

When the person who can decide is deeply committed, rapid progress may be possible. In Uruguay, starting in 2005, President Tabaré Vázquez implemented what were then the world's best tobacco control policies. President Vázquez, an oncologist, stopped cancer not only with chemotherapy but, for many more people, with effective laws and regulations. Vázquez made all public places smoke-free before any other country in the hemisphere, increased tobacco taxes, mandated plain packaging of cigarettes, and stood up to—and defeated—the tobacco industry when they tried to block the measures. His program reduced the smoking rate by more than a third.[4]

Influence isn't only about individuals—institutions matter. A business coalition can oppose government action without harming its funders' brand.

The beverage association killed the soda tax proposal without sullying Coke or Pepsi's reputation. This is why tobacco, alcohol, beverage, and junk food companies form associations. Similarly, the US Chamber of Commerce has lobbied for the tobacco industry.[5] People advocating for healthy change need to learn this lesson and form strong associations, including strategic alliances with groups that have different priorities and values. Despite their rivalry, Coke and Pepsi collaborate to kill soda taxes. Doctors, nurses, health departments, and others must work with organizations that share specific goals. Despite the powerful interests that oppose public health action, there's a way to get the formula implemented: advocates.

ADVOCACY AND PARTNERSHIPS

The fight against tuberculosis shows how advocacy can turn diffuse benefits into focused action. In 1991, multidrug-resistant strains were spreading in New York City hospitals, homeless shelters, and jails. I was clueless about good management (as described in chapter 5) and especially about being strategic. James Q. Wilson (whose book *Bureaucracy* is surprisingly fascinating) gave advice: "Make sure you have groups outside of government pushing you to do the things you need to do. Otherwise, they won't happen, or, if they do, they won't continue when you're no longer there."

When Mayor Rudy Giuliani succeeded Mayor David Dinkins, we feared he would cut the millions of dollars we had secured to renovate the dilapidated tuberculosis clinics. After all, these funds would benefit tuberculosis patients, who are generally powerless, and the money could go to much more popular programs. A letter to the new mayor from the New York Coalition to Eliminate Tuberculosis demanded that the clinic renovation continue and produced a written response that locked the money in and saved the clinics. At that time, the coalition consisted of one member: Charles Ahlers. Ahlers, a cured tuberculosis patient, had tapped out the letter on his manual typewriter. A quotation attributed to Margaret Mead highlights the importance of advocates: "Never doubt that a small group of thoughtful, committed citizens can change the world; indeed, it's the only thing that ever has."

Public health agencies and organizations are, and perhaps forever will be, underfunded, with insufficient power and authority to protect and improve health. Advocates and advocacy organizations are essential for all aspects of the See/Believe/Create formula, particularly for neglected issues and underserved populations. Activists can show health threats and progress and can pressure and support government to protect the public's health. Advocates are especially important to counteract powerful economic interests such as the tobacco industry.

Matt Myers spent forty years fighting the tobacco industry and usually winning. In Vermont, during the push for a statewide smoke-free law, one legislator had the swing vote. Myers visited the hapless politician in his office the day before the vote and laid two full-page ads for the state's leading newspaper in front of him. In one, the ad thanked the legislator for protecting Vermont's children. In the other, Vermonters held the legislator responsible for getting their children hooked on and dying from tobacco. "Assemblyman," Myers explained, "one of these two full-page ads is definitely running tomorrow. You get to choose which by how you vote today." The legislator voted for the measure, and Vermont's workplaces, government buildings, restaurants, and schools became smoke-free.

People who are directly affected can be the most persuasive advocates.[6] When the New York City Council considered the law to make restaurants and bars smoke-free, a pregnant waitress, Martinah Payne-Yehuda, joined the opening panel along with Mayor Bloomberg, Nobel Laureate Harold Varmus, and me.[7] City Council leaders later told me that the waitress's testimony was by far the most powerful: There simply is no answer to why she had to continue to be exposed and risk her pregnancy so people could smoke in her workplace.

But even with the most effective advocacy, success can be elusive. The intricate details of legislation show why politics is an art.

PRAGMATISM AND TIMING

Joe Cherner worked for years to reduce tobacco use in New York City. At age thirty, he had made enough money as a bond trader on Wall Street to retire and devote himself to strategic advocacy. Before the 2001 election for mayor and City Council, his organization (BREATHE—Bar and Restaurant Employees Advocating Together for a Healthy Environment, which consisted primarily of him) sent a survey to every mayoral and City Council candidate requesting their position on smoke-free workplaces, including restaurants and bars. We were optimistic: Bloomberg was committed to public health and most city councilmembers had committed, in signed questionnaires that Cherner posted on his website, to make New York City public places smoke-free.

It soon became clear that including restaurants in the law would be controversial, and smoke-free bars seemed out of the question. During negotiations, Cherner recommended that, if necessary, we could compromise and accept a law that would ban smoking in most places, including restaurants, and ban smoking in bars three years later. He reasoned—understanding how to use hyperbolic discounting in our favor—that people wouldn't focus on something that wouldn't happen until years into the future. But when we met with Bloomberg, he said simply, "Nothing doing. If secondhand smoke is killing people today, we ban it today. No delay for bars."

There was just one problem. Despite compelling testimony from the waitress Martinah Payne-Yehuda and other workers, the speaker of the City Council blocked the law: He refused to pass a law without allowing separate smoking rooms. If bars build separate smoking rooms, it's difficult or impossible to pass a stricter law to get rid of them. Smoking rooms undermine the benefit of smoke-free laws: Smokers continue to smoke and to expose workers. In political negotiations, knowing when to compromise is an art; this was not a compromise we could agree to, because it would make the law ineffectual. It seemed as if our highest-priority initiative, one launched with great fanfare (including a press conference that included, implausibly, New York Mets pitcher Al Leiter and Reverend Calvin Butts) would fail.

Cherner came up with the outline of a solution: Amend the proposed law to allow bars to have separate smoking rooms, but make the rooms hard to build and allow them to operate for only three years, after which the rooms would have to close. Tuberculosis isolation rooms showed the way: They're difficult and expensive to build. We wrote the legislation so bars could indeed have separate smoking rooms, but these rooms had to be at negative pressure relative to the rest of the bar, have six air changes per hour, and exhaust air through a separate system, with the exhaust pipe at least six feet from any air intake. The health department would have to approve the engineering plans and inspect the room to confirm it met the requirements. To protect workers, there could be no food or drink service in the rooms. And the rooms would have to close in three years. The speaker met his commitment to a donor who had insisted on separate smoking rooms and the legislation went through without a compromise that would have undermined it. I had learned more about that combination of science and politics my father had identified decades earlier. Two bars considered building smoking rooms; after understanding the requirements, none did.

Like politics, public health is the art of the possible; getting the timing right is one component of that art. The day after the City Council approved Mayor Bloomberg's smoking ban, the mayor and his cabinet met and Bloomberg asked me, "What's next?" I didn't have the faintest idea—I hadn't even begun to think about the next initiative. Sitting in my direct line of sight but out of the mayor's, Peter Madonia, the mayor's chief of staff, held out his left arm and pantomimed shooting up. I blurted out, "Needle exchange programs!" Months earlier, Madonia had asked me about thorny public health issues; two New York City boroughs, Queens and Staten Island, needed syringe exchange programs, but this had been politically untenable. Now, with the go-ahead from Bloomberg, we met with community boards in those boroughs and provided facts, including testimony of women infected by partners they hadn't known were at risk for HIV; the boards approved the new programs nearly unanimously.

Madonia explained an essential dictum of politics: Do the hard things first. Like a new car that loses value the moment it's driven off a sales lot, a new political administration rapidly loses political capital. It was early in the Mayor's first term; by implementing controversial but effective programs quickly, the benefits of these programs were clear and harder to reverse before the next election.

Progress requires seeing which battles are winnable, then developing and implementing a strategic plan. Years of networking and cultivation of potential allies can result in sudden opportunities for progress. An election may bring new leaders, some of whom public health staff have worked with for years. As a result, overnight a legislative or administrative measure may go from being unthinkable to inevitable. The opposite also occurs as leadership of government and organizations change. The window of opportunity for policy change can open and shut rapidly. Changing administrations, even within the same political party, present opportunities and risks to programs, personnel, and policies.

Only governments can reach entire societies, but government action is slow, and powerful forces oppose public health. A critical triad makes progress possible: strong government, proactive civil society, and rigorous monitoring to keep everyone on track. The most effective public health programs are implemented by a strong public sector, held accountable by community organizations and passionate advocates, and ensure objective monitoring.[8] Monitoring helps protect programs from budget cuts, political interference, and administrative undermining. When monitoring reveals that programs are failing, civil society groups and reform-minded government staff can intervene. Advocates can make or break programs and sustain them.

But to implement programs, it's necessary to understand and navigate not only political but also economic interests.

COMMERCIAL INTERESTS

The odds don't favor public health: Rich and powerful industries and economic interests harmful to health on one side and underfunded public health programs on the other. Implementing the formula requires tipping both sides of that scale toward health.

The profit motive drives efficiency, innovation, and consumer choice but doesn't inherently protect or improve health. Some powerful, profitable industries fight against public health progress. Industry can block or support each part of the formula—undermining efforts to see the invisible, believe that change is possible, and do what's needed to create a healthier future. The spectrum of commercial interests ranges from inherently hostile to companies whose economic incentives align with public health.

The tobacco, alcohol, junk food, gun, fossil fuel, and other industries try to sabotage each part of the formula. To prevent us from seeing, they hide the harms of their products and obscure the path to progress by funding misleading research and trying to infiltrate public health institutions and weaken guidance.[9] To block belief in change, they strengthen the illusion that use of their products is a normal part of life and that climate change, cancers, heart attacks, and other harms their products cause are inevitable. To block solutions, they lobby against effective actions such as taxation, regulation, and restrictions on marketing, sales, and promotion. They hide their activities with donations to and engagement with community groups and governments, depicting themselves as protecting the health that their actions undermine. The mandate of public health is clear: Tax and otherwise restrict these products and limit the ability of the companies that make them to obstruct public understanding and action. There's been progress on tobacco, with a global treaty and progress in more than a hundred countries, but the battle is far from won; tobacco use kills 8 million people every year.

Other industries can cause harm through their production or commercial activities unless government oversees them effectively. Dr. Alice Hamilton demonstrated the need for worker protection laws. Health departments monitor restaurants to prevent food poisoning, and the federal government regulates pharmaceutical companies to prevent fatal contamination. Environmental controls reduce factory pollution. With appropriate regulation, these industries can contribute to rather than harm health.

Further along the spectrum are entities whose products can be harmful or helpful depending on whether and how government regulates. Infant formula is essential for growth and survival of some premature infants and for other children, but irresponsible marketing has caused infant deaths around the world. Pesticides and fertilizers can increase crop yields and prevent starvation but they can poison workers and residents, contaminate soil and water, damage ecosystems, and reduce biodiversity. Dietary supplements can improve health, but marketing unproven or useless products wastes money and may steer people away from life-saving treatment.

Health-related industries are a special, and especially complicated, case. For vaccines, governments often fund research and development, train clinicians, educate the public, and buy billions of doses. The appropriate role of vaccine manufacturers is to produce safe and effective vaccines and support the research to document that they have done so. Vaccine recommendations need to be made—always and only—by individuals and entities with no financial interest in the recommendation being followed.

Regulation of medications, beyond safety and efficacy, depends on the legal and political context. Safe and effective medications that are affordable, available, and promoted responsibly can improve health. Although the pharmaceutical industry argues against mandated price reductions, claiming its profits enable life-saving research, most profits go to activities other than research.[10] Regulation, including to restrict unwarranted claims and the promotion of unproven or unnecessarily expensive medications, has the potential to increase access to medications and the affordability of health care while not harming innovation.

In health care, concentrated forces—specialists and hospitals—skew priorities and block improvements in primary care. Prevention and primary care reach more people but lack influential advocates; specialists are more prominent, and medical equipment manufacturers and other powerful interests lobby for hospitals. Some health systems succeed: Kaiser Permanente's incentives favor prevention; Costa Rica and Thailand have built strong primary care networks. But concentrated interests often block efforts to strengthen essential care. In the epilogue, we'll see how to overcome these challenges.

Some businesses contribute to health progress. Economic progress reduces poverty, the strongest predictor of ill health. Jobs improve family income and health. These are health-promoting economic activities and are at the base of the health impact pyramid (figure 3.1). New technologies can make health programs more efficient and effective. Media companies can publicize impending threats, educational companies can improve student outcomes, gyms and equipment manufacturers can increase physical activity, and companies can sell healthy food, such as potassium-enriched low-sodium salt.

Public-private partnerships can achieve more than either sector can alone. Pharmaceutical companies have sponsored well-structured medication donation programs such as those to fight river blindness, end blinding trachoma, and eradicate guinea worm; these programs have protected tens of millions of people from suffering.[11] Global vaccine programs benefit from public procurement and private production. Many sectors promote health indirectly, such as by improving roads, digital connectivity, water, and sanitation. In many of these, sensible regulations and appropriate economic incentives can make private enterprises profitable and also health-promoting.

Tipping the balance toward health requires understanding how each industry or company affects the formula: whether people see future harms, believe progress is possible, and take action. Working with political leaders and the court system, public health has powerful tools, ranging from media attention to taxation, regulation, bans, and litigation.[12] The profit motive isn't inherently inimical to health—it's generally oblivious to it. Public health can encourage industries that promote health and restrict those that harm health—but only if it has adequate funding.

FUNDING PUBLIC HEALTH

During an event at the elegant Naval Observatory, then–Vice President Joe Biden shouted, "Tom Frieden of the CDC! Thank you for protecting us." I smiled, until his next shout-out: "Francis Collins of the NIH. We're going to send you a lot more money, man!" The NIH, which supports important basic research, is not involved in the implementation of public health programs.

The Cassandra that is public health isn't just ignored—it's also broke. Health departments can't create a healthy future on a shoestring; budgets set the boundaries of the possible. Hermann Biggs, who ran the New York City and New York State Health departments at the turn of the twentieth century, had a dictum: "Public health is purchasable. Within natural limitations, a community can determine its own death rate."[13]

Public health programs—and the people who rely on them—live or die based on budgets. Many benefits won't accrue for years—until well after the next election cycle, and not to those who fund the programs. When an initiative helps smokers quit, reduced health care costs save health insurers many times the cost of the program. But savings go to the wrong pocket—the costs from the threadbare public health pocket and the benefits into the already-stuffed health insurance industry pockets.

Senator Daniel Inouye was a legend, a World War II hero who earned a Medal of Honor for exceptional bravery. He led his platoon even after being shot in the stomach and losing his right arm to a grenade. He went on to become one of the most powerful people in Washington. As chair of the Senate Appropriations Committee, he had even more say than the president in allocating money. The CDC's budget was insufficient, and I had no idea how we would protect people without more resources. Our once-world-leading labs were falling far behind. I asked Senator Inouye for advice. How could we get funding for programs that would save lives? In a slow, measured voice, he responded: "Don't tell us about the good things that will happen if we give you the money. Tell us about the bad things that will happen—*to us*—if we don't give you the money." This is the *See* part of the formula: Show legislators the harms of their actions or inaction.

The United States government's budget has followed a complicated path. First, specialists who understand what's needed make a proposal within their agency. Many offices review the proposal, cutting it deeply. Then the request leaves the agency to battle with many truly wonderful programs in other agencies. What's more important, Early Head Start or ventilators for a crisis that may not happen? Community clinics or a vaccine for a strain of influenza that may never spread? Research to end HIV, Alzheimer's, or cancer, or funds to find and stop the next pandemic that could kill millions of Americans? The proposal is cut again.

But it doesn't stop there. Even if the budget to protect Americans from deadly health threats makes it through this gauntlet, traditionally, all budget proposals take a trip to the Office of Management and Budget at the White House or the equivalent in other governments. There, smart young staffers make balance sheets add up while cutting as little as possible from politically sensitive programs; they slash the proposal more. Then . . . it goes to Congress, which generally ignores the now-decimated request and bases this year's budget on a slight adjustment of last year's budget. This is known as the "budget dance."

Consider the genomic sequencing technology that cracked the case of how tuberculosis spread, described in chapter 1. By 2010, CDC laboratories, once world-leading, had fallen far behind: Some high school labs had more advanced molecular biology capacities than the agency entrusted with protecting Americans' health. Scientists documented the need for a $200 million annual program to upgrade the labs. After the budget dance, the budget office reduced the request to $30 million. CDC received the $30 million—about one-seventh of what was needed—only after dozens of meetings with Congress and a major push from advocates inside and outside government. When COVID hit, this funding had laid the groundwork for the genomic sequencing and wastewater surveillance that made it possible to track and respond more effectively—although belatedly, because the approved budget had been so much lower than the amount CDC needed.

In my experience, well-conceived and well-written proposals eventually get funded, although often not at the level needed. Funding may not come easily or quickly, but at some point a catalyst makes funding possible: a political leader looks for a new area to invest in, an advocate or advocacy group influences a decision-maker, a media event draws attention to a neglected issue. Budget directors aren't just accountants; most want to see positive impacts of allocated funds. A cogent proposal can make funding much more likely. Progress may take years, but that's no reason to work slowly: The opportunity could arise tomorrow and fade the next day. Success requires tracking the context to see when, how, and by whom policies can be advanced.

When Mayor Bloomberg ran for reelection in 2005, he was making campaign promises; it was a great time to propose a new program. We wanted to improve health care in New York City's poorest and sickest neighborhoods—the South Bronx, Harlem, and Central Brooklyn—by providing prevention-oriented electronic health records. Learning that the mayor would make a speech on health the following week, on Friday afternoon I called a contact at the city's Office of Management and Budget, which would have to approve the proposal, and pitched the idea. Over the weekend, we designed a $27 million proposal for an election promise: The city budget would cover the costs of implementing the electronic records program in the neighborhoods that could benefit most. The mayor announced the program that week. Over the following years, doctors serving these communities got electronic health records and their patients got better care.[14]

Even fiscal austerity creates opportunities. "Revenue hunger," as economists describe limited government funding, makes it more likely government will tax tobacco, alcohol, sugary beverages, and other junk food. Public awareness can also create windows of opportunity. Media coverage ranging from celebrity illnesses to tragic preventable deaths can lead to public health funding. Similarly, recognition of positive and negative health trends creates opportunities to fund new programs. Sometimes it takes a crisis to catalyze progress. The increase in overdose deaths in the United States enables funding for programs, such as wider availability of methadone and buprenorphine and safe injection spaces, that were unthinkable previously.

The United States spends at least 300 times more on our military defense than on our health defense, yet COVID killed more than a million Americans—more than any war in our history and more than all wars since the Civil War combined. Funds for health protection are little more than a rounding error on health care costs. In a crisis, Congress can usually be convinced to provide one-time, supplemental funding, as it did for the H1N1 influenza, Ebola, Zika, and COVID emergencies. This funding is exempt from budget caps. But supplemental funding responds to an emergency and doesn't allow long-term hiring, contracting, or partnerships with organizations and countries to prevent or stop the next emergency. Unless Congress creates a new mechanism, funding to protect Americans from health threats is likely to remain unreliable. A proposed funding mechanism—termed Health Defense Operations—could put health protection on stable financial footing. Congress would allocate funds for specific health defense budget lines without reducing funds for other programs, and would oversee these programs.[15] With bipartisan support and pressure from advocates inside and outside government, the proposal could become law.

Nonprofit groups also face challenges getting adequate funding. Government funding may reduce an organization's credibility but can be essential for organizational survival.[16] Such funding can work well if the government and the group have the same interests and the government doesn't impose unwarranted restrictions on what the group can say, purchase, or do. Donations from the public and foundations can provide support; ultimately, every organization needs sufficient funding or it will cease to function.

Soon after New York City raised the tobacco tax in 2002, smuggling became a problem. Higher taxes increase the cost of cigarettes, and this induces many smokers to quit. Smuggling cheap cigarettes cuts city revenues, reduces the cost of cigarettes, and undermines the incentive to quit. The city's finance commissioner, Martha Stark, had the power to enforce the tax, and doing so would reduce smoking. Finance commissioners outrank health commissioners—money talks—so I was nervous asking her to take on cigarette smuggling. We worked hard and prepared an analysis that showed that in addition to reducing smoking, enforcement would increase the city's tax revenues by $50 million. To a health commissioner, that's a lot of money. Stark listened intently, then said, "I collect $18 billion a year in revenue. Another $50 million is hardly worth my picking up the phone. But nothing else I do will save thousands of lives. I'll do it."

Public health actions are often cost-effective.[17] A few initiatives, such as sodium reduction, save money.[18] But financial savings don't get policies implemented, and many programs don't save money. The tobacco industry unintentionally demonstrated why focusing on financial savings from public health action is wrong. Hoping to stop regulations in the Czech Republic, they published a study that showed that countries save money from smokers who die young and thus don't collect their pensions, housing, and other benefits.[19] The publication backfired; as an actuary friend commented, "From that argument to 'mortality risk-adjustment squads' is a thin line." The regulations passed. Although governments might spend less on people who die young, successful public health programs decrease disability, reduce annual health care costs, and increase productivity. The fundamental goal of public health is to save lives, not to save money.

Tobacco taxation increases government revenues, reduces per capita health expenditures, saves lives, and has many other health benefits, but less than 15 percent of people in the world live in areas with effective tobacco taxation. This isn't because finance ministers are foolish, but because tobacco companies are powerful.

Geoffrey Rose puts the relationship between economics and health into perspective:

> Prevention of deaths is only likely to involve net economic advantage if it applies to children or young adults, and beyond the age of about 50 the economic outcome is increasingly negative as applied to preventive measures which extend survival. However, at every age before retirement there is an economic gain from any preventive policy which can reduce disability or improve working capacity, and after retirement there are economic savings from anything which enhances independence and reduces the need for medical and social supports.
>
> It is better to be healthy than ill or dead. That is the beginning and the end of the only real argument for preventive medicine. It is sufficient.[20]

Although health may, as Rose wrote, be a sufficient ethical argument, it's only by getting strategy, advocacy, partnerships, and messaging right that healthy policies get enacted.

Tipping the balance to manage commercial interests and increase funding for public health is hard, but the issues are straightforward. A more complex political question to navigate is when public health should exercise its "police powers."

PUBLIC HEALTH LAW

To manage the political and economic forces that block life-saving actions, public health agencies have a powerful—but increasingly controversial—tool: regulation. This authority allowed us to figure out, in 1991, that drug-resistant tuberculosis was increasing and spreading in New York City hospitals. Health departments require restaurants to operate in sanitary ways, childcare providers to serve safe and healthy food, and doctors to report infectious diseases. Laws—the lightning Bloomberg described with the quotation from Mark Twain—can protect health.

For several years in the early 1990s, Angel, an inaptly named tuberculosis patient, had been admitted to—and then, against medical advice, signed out from—hospitals throughout New York City more than thirty times. He would feel better after a few weeks, stop taking treatment, and become highly infectious. As a result, his tuberculosis strain had become resistant to nearly every medication. Angel personified three aspects of the tuberculosis resurgence: the increase in drug resistance Karen Brudney had seen, the hospital spread that genomic epidemiology revealed, and the central importance of tracking every patient's care as Karel Styblo advised.

Public fear was intense. Doctors in training avoided New York City hospitals because they feared infection with multidrug-resistant tuberculosis. HIV was spreading widely, making the threat even more serious. Tabloid headlines demanded the city jail tuberculosis patients. Some activists opposed all mandates, pointing out that tuberculosis isn't a crime. Meanwhile, the communities most affected by tuberculosis were clear: At a public meeting in Harlem, the audience was unanimous. "Why didn't you lock up tuberculosis patients who don't take their medicine years ago, before it got this bad?" The city found a middle ground. Rather than jailing patients, we created a range of interventions, starting with positive incentives—food, vouchers, and social support, including housing. We took the least restrictive alternative that could succeed, starting with mandatory outpatient care. This worked for most patients who had stopped treatment. When necessary, after assessing each patient individually, we detained patients, not in a jail but in specially designed secure hospital units. We provided legal representation and periodic judicial review for every detained patient. Although this restricted the liberty of patients (139 out of more than 8,000—less than 2 percent—in the first two years of the program), it prevented thousands of infections and saved lives.[21]

Boston's tuberculosis detention coordinator, who operated a similar program for years, explained their pragmatic perspective:

> When we admit patients, they are often homeless, addicted to drugs or alcohol, mentally ill, HIV-infected and have tuberculosis. We do whatever we can, but the plain truth is that when they leave, most will still be homeless, addicted to drugs or alcohol, mentally ill, and HIV positive. But they won't have tuberculosis, and that's a big deal for them and for their family and community.

Although some patients died from AIDS, for which effective treatment hadn't yet been discovered, the New York City program cured nearly all detained patients.[22] Angel's strain had become resistant to almost all antibiotics, and tuberculosis had destroyed his lungs; by the time we detained him, even the best care couldn't cure his infection. Failing to ensure treatment not only endangered health care workers and communities—it killed Angel.

Legal measures aren't always the answer, as the 2014–2016 West African Ebola epidemic showed. When I met with President Alpha Conde of Guinea, he was understandably frustrated and literally shaking with anger: Guinea received far less support than the other countries affected by the epidemic even though it's bigger and has a larger population. President Conde wanted to force communities to close so exposed contacts couldn't travel and trigger new clusters of Ebola. I urged him instead to expand services to affected communities. "There's a saying," I said, "that you catch more flies with honey than with vinegar." "Yes," Conde replied quickly, "but the honey has to get there before the flies leave!"

President Conde was right, as a distressing insight from Dr. Abdou Salam Gueye showed. Dr. Gueye is a Senegalese physician epidemiologist CDC sent to Guinea for months at the height of the Ebola epidemic. He had completed the CDC's Epidemic Intelligence Service training and combined deep knowledge of the region with epidemiologic expertise. He summarized: "Do you know what people in the communities are saying about the CDC teams? 'You say you're doctors, but you've been here for eighteen months and you haven't treated a single patient.'" This was painful to hear. CDC had been so focused on infection control, contact tracing, and stopping outbreaks it had neglected community concerns and the importance of earning the community's trust.

Fortunately, there was a way to act on this insight. Faced with continued outbreaks of Ebola in rural villages, in June 2015, public health leaders in Guinea created a strategy that became a best practice: *microcerclage*—microencirclement. When a community reported a case of Ebola, authorities restricted travel: People could leave, but because they might need to be traced if they had been in contact with an Ebola patient, they were required to provide their cell phone number, where they were going, and when they would return. The government provided comprehensive support: doctors and nurses who gave childhood vaccinations and other health care; food, antimalarial bed nets, and soap; and community education.[23] Doctors evaluated everyone who developed symptoms of Ebola and provided care quickly. The strategy worked: Nearby communities without Ebola cases asked if they, too, could undergo microcerclage.

For the entire epidemic, Sierra Leone didn't learn this lesson and insisted on posting police outside the houses of named contacts of Ebola cases. This led to stigma, bribery, and avoidable hardship. Police prevented people who had been identified as contacts from planting or harvesting their crops; contacts of cases saw planting season come and go and faced a year of hunger and hardship. The result? People didn't trust government, patients didn't name contacts, and these contacts developed and spread Ebola. The Sierra Leone Ebola epidemic continued for many months longer than it would have without this unnecessarily harsh response.

The legal framework for contact tracing and quarantine is a small but essential part of public health practice. It relies on political support for public health and, if done well, prevents clusters from becoming outbreaks and outbreaks from becoming epidemics.[24] But there's a balance between individual rights and public protection. When are mandates justified?

THE MANDATE FOR MANDATES

We have long accepted regulations that allow public health agencies to track and control tuberculosis, Ebola, and other infectious diseases. Most people would agree that if it's the only way to prevent spread of multidrug-resistant tuberculosis, long-term hospital detention of patients like Angel—after due process—is appropriate. Although wearing a face mask can be inconvenient and uncomfortable and reduces communication, it's hardly in the same category as compulsory confinement. Why, if forcible detention of tuberculosis patients is acceptable, were mask mandates and other requirements so controversial during the COVID pandemic?

The principle of tuberculosis detention is straightforward: Just as your right to swing your fist ends at my nose, your right to skip medications doesn't extend to coughing multidrug-resistant tuberculosis into my lungs. But the rationale for COVID-related mandates isn't as clear.

Start with mask mandates. COVID can spread before people feel sick, so wearing a mask only when you're ill isn't sufficient; if everyone wears a mask indoors when COVID is spreading widely, everyone will be safer. The defensibility of a mask mandate depends on context. Everyone who enters a hospital unit for children receiving chemotherapy should be required to use a mask. No one outside in open space should be required to do so. Between these extremes, many considerations will determine whether and when a mask mandate is appropriate. How much COVID is spreading? How transmissible is the current variant? How deadly? Are vaccines available and effective? Treatments? How many medically vulnerable people may get infected? Will hospitals become overwhelmed? What does the community value most? It's unfortunate that mask-wearing became partisan and polarizing. If someone is violently sick with infectious diarrhea, they shouldn't refuse to wash their hands and then prepare food for others. Like handwashing, indoor mask-wearing reduces harm to others.

Business closure mandates are much more extreme. Unlike prohibiting food contamination in restaurants, closing businesses affects livelihoods and economic stability. Although closures protect workers from infection and reduce the risk that COVID patients will overwhelm hospitals, they're only justifiable if the health and societal benefits outweigh the harms, there is no realistic less restrictive alternative, and the affected community participates in the decision process. As tuberculosis treatment programs and Ebola responses showed, mandates work best when they start with positive support, escalate only when necessary and with clear communication of the justification, and maintain community trust.

An effective approach to decisions about mandates is to define objective risk-alert levels—essentially, how hard it's raining COVID in an area and whether the health system is or may soon become overwhelmed.[25] As with ozone, fire, and hurricane warning systems, risk-alert levels empower individuals and communities to choose appropriate protective actions. At the "all clear" level (green), no mandates are indicated. At the "some risk" level (yellow), there are no mandates, but vulnerable people and others who are concerned may decide to limit activities or wear a mask, as people with asthma may when informed that ozone levels are high.[26] When COVID is spreading widely and it's "high risk" (orange), some communities may mandate mask-wearing indoors and close restaurants, bars, and other indoor, in-person businesses. Different choices in different communities are appropriate; communities will need to comply with mandates, so people should understand the risks, benefits, and data supporting the risk-alert level, and be part of the decision-making process. At the highest risk level (red), with extensive spread and health care systems potentially overwhelmed, more restrictive policies such as indoor mask mandates are indicated: Mandates that decrease disease spread help prevent broad harms. This is analogous to a ban on starting campfires in a parched forest.

Some vaccine mandates are particularly controversial. Requiring students to get vaccinated as a condition of school entry increases vaccination coverage and can reduce the spread of measles, pertussis, meningitis, and other diseases.[27] Parents who don't vaccinate their child put other children—particularly those with a medical condition that makes them vulnerable—at risk. COVID vaccination mandates proved much more complex. Initial COVID vaccine trial results suggested that vaccination prevented infection. At that time, few people had immunity and COVID killed approximately 1 in 200 people it infected and a much higher proportion of the elderly. The combination of a vaccine that prevented infection and therefore protected others plus the high mortality rate made vaccine mandates appear justified.

As more data became available and new variants emerged, it became clear that the vaccine's ability to prevent infection and therefore protect others wanes within several months (protection from severe illness and death lasts longer). This information weakened the case for a broad public mandate; mandates are most defensible when vaccination protects others. Furthermore, as vaccination and infection increased the proportion of people with immunity and treatment improved, the virus became less lethal, killing approximately 1 in 1,000 people infected, with mortality rates as low as 1 in 10,000 or lower among younger people up to date with vaccines. This further weakened the case for a mandate.[28]

With emerging scientific data about the vaccine and increasing population immunity, COVID vaccination mandates turned out to be closer to motorcycle helmet laws than school vaccine requirements. Helmet laws benefit society by reducing medical, rehabilitation, and disability costs, but their main purpose is to protect the rider. Similarly, COVID vaccine mandates reduce infections and broader societal harms somewhat, but the major benefit is to the vaccinated person. Adults can choose to risk their own safety—for example, by smoking, participating in extreme sports, or cave diving—as long as they don't harm others. Because COVID vaccination mandates, like helmet laws, primarily protect the person mandated, decisions are best made at the state and local level. This allows for public debate, transparent decision-making, and—if mandates are enacted—better compliance.

To regain trust, mandates must be rare, appropriate, specific to time and place, and updated as we learn more. Technical agencies face an inherent tension between professional standards and political realities.[29] They must bridge gaps between politics and science, theory and practice, and community and individual incentives. Governments may ignore public health recommendations that don't account for context and feasibility, and the public isn't likely to trust recommendations that are seen as politically motivated.[30] Either extreme—too rigid or too political—can cost lives. The failure of Prohibition shows that even well-intentioned policies collapse without public support.

Mandates are just one type of law to promote health. When are other legal actions justifiable to stop health threats, including today's leading killers: tobacco, air pollution, alcohol, and obesity?

NANNY STATE OR RESPONSIVE GOVERNMENT?

"Nanny State!" the tabloids blared when New York City made bars and restaurants smoke-free, banned trans fat, and mandated calorie counts on menu boards. Do taxation, regulation, and bans infantilize adults and overreach government's appropriate role?[31]

There have been allegations of public health overreach for more than a century. In the 1890s, the New York State Medical Society attacked the requirement that doctors report tuberculosis cases to public health authorities as "mistaken, untimely, irrational and unwise" and tried to have the measure revoked.[32]

The nanny state critique misses the invisible forces that influence decisions. Behavior reflects not just personal choices but also economic, social, and political context. Differences in self-control don't explain why rates of smoking, obesity, and drug use are wildly different in different places and change over time. The context—price, accessibility, marketing, and social norms—determines use rates. By mitigating these external forces, public health *increases* individuals' control over their health and life. Government action can make the healthier choice easier.

Actions that were once controversial—banning the sale of contaminated food, outlawing ads for useless medicine, and reducing drunk driving—are now widely accepted. These examples illustrate three justifiable public health strategies. The first is health protection—protecting people from harms, whether from contaminated food or untreated tuberculosis. This is no more "nanny state" than preventing assault and homicide. The second is providing information, which empowers people to make more informed choices about their health. The third is collective action, which addresses the unavoidable interdependence of modern society and can promote health more effectively and efficiently than individual effort. (See table 8.1 for traditional and newer examples of each.) We can't stay safe when contaminated food, water, and addictive substances pervade our community. Community-wide action that protects our food, work, and environment helps everyone thrive.

Although no state in the US has passed a soda tax, more than forty cities and more than thirty countries, from Mexico to the United Kingdom to Malaysia, have done so. Evidence for the benefits of soda taxes is strong: These taxes generate substantial revenue, reduce soda consumption, and are likely to improve health.[33] Children in cities with soda taxes appear to have lower rates of obesity.[34] Sometimes, it's important not just to have the right issue, strategy, messages, and timing but also to choose the right

Table 8.1

Public health actions of a responsive government

Protecting people from harm they can't control—from others, pathogens, or nature	Promoting free and open information	Taking societal action to protect and promote health
Long-standing		
Prevention of food adulteration	Truth-in-advertising laws	School vaccination mandates
Laws against alcohol-impaired driving	Nutrition-facts panel	Micronutrient fortification of
Infectious disease reporting	Pharmaceutical package	manufactured foods (e.g.,
Worker safety	inserts	iodization of salt)
Protection against naturally occurring health threats (e.g., West Nile virus)		Clean water, air, food
Tobacco excise tax		Elimination of lead from paint and gasoline
Alcohol excise tax		
Newer		
Laws requiring smoke-free workplaces and other public places	Public reporting of health care provider performance	Zoning laws to promote physical activity (e.g., paths for walking and bicycling)
Alcohol ignition interlock devices for people convicted of drunk driving	Calorie and sodium labeling at chain restaurants	School policies (e.g., food, physical activity, safe transportation)
Restrictions on sale and marketing of tobacco and alcohol (especially to children)	Graphic tobacco pack warnings	Reduction of sodium in packaged and restaurant foods
Elimination of artificial trans fat		

Source: Thomas R. Frieden, "Government's Role in Protecting Health and Safety," *New England Journal of Medicine* 368, no. 20 (May 16, 2013): 1857–1859.

battleground. On some controversial issues, most states in the US are simply too vulnerable to commercial interests to make much progress.

Passing soda taxes required getting every aspect of the formula right (see appendix 1 for a ready-reference guide). See: The superpower of surveillance showed that sugar-sweetened beverages are the single largest driver of increased calorie consumption. Believe: The effectiveness of tobacco and alcohol taxes bolstered confidence that soda taxes would be effective. Create: A strategic, well-communicated political strategy countered each of the forces that blind us to Cassandra-like warnings. Advocates explained a simple truth: Liquid calories don't satisfy hunger. Eating a chocolate bar spoils your appetite; drinking a soda doesn't. Mike Bloomberg's philanthropy countered the economic force of soda industry lobbying with support for most of the successful efforts to increase soda taxes in the US and globally.

Framing the issue, accurately, as creating environments that make healthy choices easier shifted the narrative away from the nanny state critique. To combat the normalcy bias, advocates showed that the high level of soda consumption today is abnormal compared with that of every prior generation. Diverse coalitions that included teachers, doctors, nurses, and community organizations shifted social norms. And to address hyperbolic discounting, advocates highlighted immediate benefits, such as funding for education—Philadelphia earmarked revenue from soda taxes for early childhood programs—making benefits tangible.[35]

Part I of this book reveals the public health superpower of surveillance to *see* invisible harms, program performance, and pathways to progress. Part II shows how to help communities *believe* in the possibility of progress: highlight past progress, make further progress, and cultivate optimism. Part III shows how organization, simple and scalable solutions, and effective communication are essential to the *create* component of the formula. The current chapter outlines the importance of avoiding a naïve appeal to political will and using a rigorous analysis of interests, allies, and timing to counter the political and economic forces that block health progress.[36] So, using the formula to *see*, *believe*, and *create*, what can a healthy future look like?

PART IV THE FORMULA IN PRACTICE

9 THE FORMULA FOR PUBLIC HEALTH

The best way to predict the future is to create it.
—attributed to Peter Drucker

Imagine a joyous, healthy birth. A thriving infancy with only minor infections. All developmental milestones met during childhood. As a young adult, normal weight, good sleep and physical activity habits, a preference for healthy foods, and free from addiction to drugs, tobacco, and alcohol. Aging, no major illnesses, injuries, or disruption from a pandemic. In later years, no elevation of blood pressure, hearing loss, or major decline in mental faculties. A gentle slowing, with a peaceful death at age 103. Sounds utopian, but it's within reach if we implement the See/Believe/Create formula.

THE HEALTH OF PUBLIC HEALTH

The COVID pandemic killed 20 million people, cost more than $20 trillion, left hundreds of millions of children behind in their education, and caused widespread disability from long COVID.[1] This devastation was not inevitable; it resulted from a series of failures—to see the impending disaster and path to mitigation, believe we could control it, and create simple, scaled responses to make the pandemic less disruptive. Will we do better next time? If we spend less than one-tenth of 1 percent of the cost of COVID each year, we can protect the world against the health and economic losses of a future pandemic.[2]

As with the 1918 influenza pandemic, memory of COVID tragedies has faded fast—collective amnesia.[3] Each of the drivers of the Cassandra curse

Table 9.1

Challenges to preventing the next pandemic: Cassandra curse drivers in action

Driver	How it undermines pandemic prevention
Prevention paradox	Large improvements are imperceptible because they result from many small steps. Specific actions don't feel urgent.
Economic forces	More visible problems with stronger political support draw attention and funding.
Myth of unfettered free will	Hubris about our ability to manage future emergencies creates resistance to collective protection measures.
False alarms	Repeated warnings dull the public and political response.
Social norms and the normalcy bias	We assume that past survival guarantees future safety, despite the deaths of 20 million people from COVID.
Hyperbolic discounting	We shortchange the future, underestimating both the likelihood and severity of pandemics—even in the wake of COVID.

(table 9.1 and appendix 1 table A1.1) undermines efforts to prevent the next pandemic. Despite these challenges, we can use the formula to reduce the risk that a pandemic emerges; find and quickly stop any potential pandemic; and manage pandemics well.

The formula works. Karen Brudney sounded the alarm about the spread of drug-resistant tuberculosis and genomic epidemiology revealed that hospitals were the main source (See), allowing us to protect health care workers and patients. Karel Styblo showed the way forward and gave confidence to implement the technical package he developed (Believe), particularly the simple focus on the outcome of every patient. The doctors we hired with "Dead Lenny's" job title provided excellent care, outreach workers used superb communication to keep patients on track, and the rare patients who required a legal mandate got treatment. Advocates protected the clinics and the program (Create).

In the six years after Dr. Brudney's warning, the number of patients with multidrug-resistant tuberculosis in New York City plummeted by more than 90 percent, saving hundreds of lives and tens of millions of dollars and stopping the largest outbreak of multidrug-resistant tuberculosis the United States has ever experienced.[4]

Technological progress gives more reason for optimism about our ability to stop pandemics and other health threats. New laboratory technologies—including rapid, low-cost genomic testing of patient specimens and of wastewater—can provide early warnings and make an impending pandemic visible sooner. New information sources and analytics, including large language models, can turn messy data into actionable information. Stopping a new microbial threat is increasingly feasible with new diagnostic, treatment, and vaccine technologies.

Communities and countries have shown they can more rapidly detect and stop outbreaks. Global collaboration can facilitate scaling solutions to entire countries, regions, and the world. Strategic communication with the right messages and messengers can enable and catalyze progress. New financing mechanisms can provide stable resources. And strong institutions can fight for, implement, and sustain protective measures.

Unfortunately, few leaders are eager to spend money, time, and attention to prevent a problem that may not happen before the next election. That's why the playbook for political progress is so important: Find and empower champions and groups within and outside government; mobilize those who win when there is effective prevention (e.g., insurance companies); and outmaneuver potential losers. Create accurate, timely, and public feedback loops to determine whether protection measures are making progress, and if not, make rapid course corrections. This is particularly important because it's certain that another pandemic will strike.

PREVENT THE NEXT PANDEMIC

A lab release or spillover from the animal world will likely cause the next pandemic; the formula shows how to prevent it. The world may never know—and almost certainly will never agree on—which of these two routes started the COVID pandemic. Microbes escape from laboratories and also emerge from contact between humans and animals. Rather than debate what caused COVID, countries and international organizations must reduce the risk of both of these routes to the next deadly pandemic.

In a little-known dirty secret, it's likely that an influenza strain that spread around the world in 1977, killing thousands of people, came from a laboratory or a botched vaccine trial, possibly from the former Soviet Union.

A review of the "Russian flu" concluded that the strain "too closely matched to decades-old strains to likely be a natural occurrence."[5] The last cases of smallpox in the world resulted from infection of a laboratory worker in the United Kingdom in 1978.[6] And in 2004, after the 2002–2003 severe acute respiratory syndrome (SARS) outbreak ended, two graduate students in China who worked with the virus in the laboratory became infected, resulting in seven additional cases, including one student's mother, who died.[7] In my time leading the CDC, although no pathogens were released and no one became infected in these incidents, by mistake live Ebola samples were sent to a less safe laboratory; a new lab instrument created a risk of anthrax exposures; a rushed lab technician accidentally sent out a dangerous strain of influenza; and the National Institutes of Health found a smallpox sample in one of their unsecured storage cabinets.[8] To err is human; to fail to plan for human error is dangerous.

Laboratories perform too many experiments, with too many dangerous pathogens, in too many institutions, staffed by too many people. The risks are high—an accidental or intentional release of a deadly pathogen could cause the next pandemic, and it could be even deadlier and costlier than COVID. Advances in biotechnology make it increasingly possible to create dangerous pathogens.

Global action can reduce risk of a laboratory release. Regulations should require that before any experiment begins, researchers make these risks visible by addressing a fundamental question: Is the potential benefit greater than the potential risk? Regulations should limit risky experiments to those with a likely substantial benefit, require organizations to reduce the number of staff and labs doing risky research, and implement and continuously improve safety policies and procedures. Implementation would require money, face resistance from researchers, and wouldn't eliminate the threat of bad actors. But until we take these steps, we're failing to heed the warnings of a future devastating human-made pandemic released from a laboratory. This is the laboratory equivalent of the prevention paradox: Each measure reduces risk only minimally, but all measures together can reduce risk substantially.[9]

These measures won't eliminate all risk. A malfunctioning exhaust hood, broken test tube, faulty centrifuge, or torn rubber glove can release pathogens. A malicious country or group—or even a smart high school student—can create a deadly pathogen with readily obtainable materials. To reduce risk, we need measures to control the availability of these materials, as specialized international agencies do for nuclear and chemical weapons. Any step that reduces risk is a step toward a safer future.

One particularly difficult challenge is regulation of so-called *gain-of-function* laboratory research—manipulation that makes an organism more contagious, more deadly, or both.[10] This includes experiments that increase the ability of deadly animal influenza viruses to spread among humans. Because of its possible dangers, there have been calls for strict regulation or banning of gain-of-function research. But gain-of-function isn't a simple on/off switch. What about engineering bacteria to produce new antibiotics? This could make these bacteria more resistant to antibiotics and therefore more likely to be lethal, but preventing such research because some gain-of-function studies are dangerous could derail efforts to treat dangerous, antibiotic-resistant microbes. The plain truth is that a wide range of research is risky. A practical approach is to apply the most stringent safeguards to the experiments that have the greatest risk of creating organisms that are particularly deadly, could spread widely, or both.

Reducing risk of spillover from animals to humans is even more challenging than reducing laboratory risk. It's a big world out there. HIV, Mpox, SARS-1, MERS (Middle East Respiratory Syndrome), multiple strains of influenza, Ebola, Marburg, and many other pathogens have spread from animals to humans on multiple continents.[11] Ebola and Marburg outbreaks may occur because of increasing human encroachment into forest areas.[12] It may be impossible to predict which microbe in which animal from which part of the world will cause the next pandemic, but we can reduce the risk of spillover.[13] If we reduce deforestation, including by supporting communities living in the forested areas, we reduce risky animal-human contacts. Brazil, with its massive Amazon Basin region, showed that progress is possible: Policies and programs implemented from 2004 to 2012 reduced the rate of deforestation by 70 percent while increasing agricultural production.[14] This improvement had major health and economic benefits but also shows how tenuous progress can be: When a subsequent government weakened policy enforcement, deforestation increased.

Wet markets sell fish, poultry, meats, and, sometimes, exotic animals. In New York City's Chinatown, I once saw a middle-aged, stone-faced grocer weigh live frogs, soon to become a frog-leg delicacy. Lightning fast, he snatched three, plopped them into a plastic bag, and nonchalantly flipped them ten feet away to the other side of the stall, where they landed, perfectly positioned, on a hanging metal spring balance, stunned momentarily as the vendor and customer agreed on the weight and price. But markets that sell live animals for food cause deadly outbreaks, especially if they sell live exotic animals. Collection and sale of "bush meat"—monkeys, bats, and other forest animals—may have spread Ebola, Lassa fever, and other deadly viruses. Search for the source of SARS-1—a coronavirus related to the COVID virus—found exotic animal markets in Guangdong Province, China where vendors sold civet cats as delicacies. These animals, which may have contracted the virus from bats, likely spread SARS-1 and triggered the global outbreak in 2002-2003.

To reduce spillover risk, we must regulate wet markets and improve the safety of raising animals for food. The limited global progress implementing these measures reflects concentrated losses (to people who operate wet markets) and diffuse benefits to people unaware of the deadly infection they would be less likely to get. Ways to reduce risk include a global, enforceable agreement to ban sale of wild animals for food, support for communities that rely on such food (including promotion of other locally available protein sources), and further progress to intensively track and reduce the risk of influenza spreading from birds, swine, and other animals to people.[15] It's not just wet markets that present a risk. The only predictable aspect of influenza is its unpredictability. Spread of influenza viruses by migratory birds, farmed animals, and people could ignite the next pandemic at any moment. Increasing our safety requires sustained funding, strengthened by advocates and institutions, along with monitoring of implementation to increase accountability.

The Burden × Amenability approach can identify the highest-risk and most controllable lab and spillover threats. The simplicity, speed, and scale approach can determine the most practical approaches and catalyze global action. Stronger national and global public health capacity to stop outbreaks will further reduce risk. Managing the challenging politics will be essential and can result in implementation of measures that will make pandemics less likely. But even with the best prevention, new threats will emerge.

FIND PANDEMICS FASTER

Making the world safer from pandemics means not only preventing them when possible but also finding and stopping them where they emerge. Chapter 5 discussed incident management systems, the essential organizational structure to manage epidemics. Chapter 6 showed how important speed is and how the 7-1-7 target can accelerate progress.

Making the world safer from infectious diseases requires global commitment and increased financing. The argument is compelling: The annual cost is less than one-tenth of 1 percent of a future pandemic's cost. Logic rarely wins political or funding arguments, but programs that increase the proportion of outbreaks that meet the 7-1-7 target can reduce disease and economic disruption and demonstrate value. Finding the necessary $5–10 billion a year requires political champions and vigorous advocacy.

Increased resources can strengthen the surveillance superpower to detect threats sooner with data from primary health care, laboratories, news and social media, wastewater, and historical and regional trends. Artificial intelligence might further strengthen predictive capacity. Faster detection can result in deployment of rapid-response teams that quickly find and stop outbreaks. Every community has strengths—respected leaders, traditions, habits, resources, organizations—and success in public health often requires identifying these strengths and enlisting them to detect or respond to an outbreak or other public health problem. In the West Africa Ebola epidemic, community leaders convinced families to modify traditional burial practices in order to reduce spread of infection. In New York City, the most effective outreach workers were recent college graduates from communities most affected by the tuberculosis outbreak. In India, tuberculosis patient supporters are community members such as child-care providers, shopkeepers, and, more recently, community health officers and activists.

Better primary health care services can improve detection of and response to health threats, but in most countries, public health and primary care are poorly connected. The alert clinician is often the most effective early-warning system—as Karen Brudney showed when she sounded the alarm about drug-resistant tuberculosis in New York City. Public health departments can inform clinicians of a potential outbreak and help doctors better diagnose and treat patients and protect themselves from infection. Primary care systems that have long-term, trusting relationships with their patients are the most effective messengers on the need for tests, treatment, and, especially, vaccinations.

It's inevitable that pandemics will occur. It's not inevitable that the response will be so delayed and ineffective that a pandemic kills millions of people. A safer future is possible—if we implement the formula. But even if the world neither prevents nor rapidly detects and stops the next pandemic, we can get better at fighting it. How? Simple: Manage a current pandemic better.

STOP A CURRENT PANDEMIC

Cholera causes severe diarrhea and dehydration, spreads rapidly, and, unless well managed, kills up to 10 percent of the people it infects. The most recent global cholera pandemic has spread since 1961–so long that we don't see it as the pandemic it is. Climate change worsens cholera by warming waters, increasing floods, reducing access to clean water, and displacing communities. Stopping the ongoing cholera pandemic would save lives, hasten economic development, and forge better mechanisms to combat future pandemics.[16]

The legendary founding moment of modern public health occurred in 1854. John Snow proved that cholera spread through contaminated water; authorities removed the handle of the Broad Street pump and ended an outbreak in London. Since then, countries around the world have built safe drinking water and sanitation systems.[17] Yet today, more than two billion people lack access to safe drinking water. In the 1990s, Peru ended its cholera epidemic by improving its water supply.[18] The world can end today's cholera pandemic with clean water, improved cholera diagnosis and treatment, and vaccination of those at risk.

Cleaner water would reduce not only cholera but also childhood deaths and adult illnesses. Better cholera diagnosis and treatment would strengthen lab networks and primary health care systems. Expanded cholera vaccination would improve global and national institutions that finance, produce, and administer vaccines—upgrading the capacity to rapidly scale up manufacturing for other vaccines as well. Managing the cholera pandemic would strengthen each aspect of the formula: surveillance to track infections and control; progress to build confidence; systematic organization for quick detection and response; improved communication with the public, medical staff, and policymakers; and strategic advocacy for funding. Success would save lives today and strengthen the systems we'll need when the next pandemic occurs.

The formula's power isn't limited to infectious diseases. Just as we often fail to see emerging pandemic threats, we overlook today's deadliest disease.

STOP THE WORLD'S DEADLIEST PANDEMIC

Public health has generally done a good job protecting people from conditions that killed people a hundred years ago. In 1900, heart disease and stroke accounted for less than one of every thirteen US deaths; they now account for nearly one of every three.[19] We are asleep at the switch to non-infectious causes of death. Hypertension, the "silent killer," is the deadliest, most neglected, and most widespread pandemic of our time. Globally, deaths from hypertension increased from 6.8 million in 1990 to nearly 11 million by 2020. Each year, hypertension kills twice as many people as the COVID pandemic did at its worst, and its victims die at a younger age than the people COVID killed. Without concerted action, the hypertension pandemic will continue to get worse and will kill more than 14 million every year by 2050. How can we apply the formula to today's leading killer?

First, see what's killing us and the status of our programs to protect ourselves. Current and future deaths are largely invisible precisely because they are so common. Heart disease and stroke are not inevitable; they result from risks we can avoid. Despite the trillions of dollars spent on health care every year, at most one in five people with hypertension in the world and half of those in the United States have it under control. Chapter 3 showed that hypertension rises to the top of the Burden × Amenability calculation and outlined the pathway forward: a technical package to make progress.

Next, strengthen the reasons to believe progress is possible. We've made enormous progress reducing cardiovascular disease, with death rates decreasing by an astonishing two-thirds from 1960 to 2010.[20] Health systems such as Kaiser Permanente and countries including Canada show that it's possible to treat the great majority of people with hypertension effectively, with success rates more than double those of average providers and countries.

To create a healthier future where heart attacks and strokes are rare, organize health care so each provider is part of a team, with nursing, social services, behavioral health, pharmacy, and community outreach. As discussed in chapter 6, establish simple diagnosis, treatment, and monitoring. Clinicians can use proven protocols to improve quality and prevent errors and give more patients better care at lower cost.[21] But, as outlined in chapter 8 and demonstrated by the failure of the Million Hearts initiative (chapter 2), success requires a fundamental change in the way we pay for health care.

A payment structure that assigns patients to specific provider teams—referred to as capitation—can reward providers when they reduce health care spending by preventing complications and hospitalizations.[22] Each team has a panel of assigned patients and is paid per patient per year, with increased or decreased payment based on health outcomes. This aligns the incentives of clinicians, patients, and the organizations that pay for care. Providers would have an incentive to establish teams that include different types of health care workers, including nurses, pharmacists, and outreach workers.

With the right incentives, providers will reduce barriers to care, for example, by refilling prescriptions automatically and ensuring medication delivery to the patient's home. Patients on stable treatment would receive three or six months of free medications. Telemedicine, email, text messages, and phone calls to address patient concerns would be easy. Doctors and others would use data—making actual performance visible—to improve outcomes continuously. Accurate information is also essential to break the inverse care law whereby people who need services most get them least.[23] The community survey in Douglas, Tennessee (chapter 7), found that higher-income people were more likely to be aware of services. By identifying groups left out, systems can restructure, reach out, and reform to care for those most in need and least likely to access services.

We pay far too much for care that does far too little to improve health and save lives. Hospitals, specialists, information systems, training programs, and insurance companies benefit from current financial incentives. In many systems, the most likely way to pay for expansion of primary care services will be to reduce unnecessary tests, hospitalizations, and services. Payors could waive copayments and deductibles for specialty visits if patients contact their primary provider first. This would reduce the excess tests, procedures, and visits that add to the cost of care yet provide little or no health benefit.

Progress becomes possible when we identify and mitigate groups with the power to veto proposed reform and the people and organizations that influence these deciders. There are policy windows—political moments when change is possible, such as when a new government comes to power, there is a budget surplus to invest or a deficit that requires reform, or when advocates, including primary care workers, insist on change. In Costa Rica, a grand bargain among all major political parties created a mandate for better health care services.[24]

For hypertension control globally, success means supporting patients, doctors, nurses, outreach workers, and country leaders so they treat at least 500 million more people effectively with safe, effective, low-cost medicines. In the United States, Medicare can establish powerful financial incentives to prevent disease. When health systems are accountable for all of their patients' medical expenses, prevention becomes profitable. Systems that prevent heart attacks, strokes, and kidney failure earn more. Those with higher rates of avoidable heart attacks, strokes, and kidney failure would face financial penalties. This would align the interest of patients in a long, healthy, disability-free life with the financial interests of the health care system and of those who pay for care.

Treatment is important, but prevention of hypertension can save at least as many lives.[25] We consume too much sodium and too little potassium.[26] Switching to potassium-enriched salt could reduce blood pressure and prevent heart attacks and strokes.[27] Reducing sodium and increasing potassium intake exemplifies the prevention paradox: Small changes can prevent large numbers of heart attacks and strokes. In the United States, the Food and Drug Administration can set, monitor, and enforce targets to reduce sodium in packaged food.[28] Stop-sign front-of-pack warnings, limits on salt quantities, taxes, and bans on marketing unhealthy foods can reduce sodium intake and hypertension.[29]

With focused effort, despite the increasing and aging global population, we can drive deaths from hypertension back below 8 million.[30] Over the next twenty-five years, this would prevent more than 50 million premature deaths and more than 100 million heart attacks and strokes (figure 9.1).

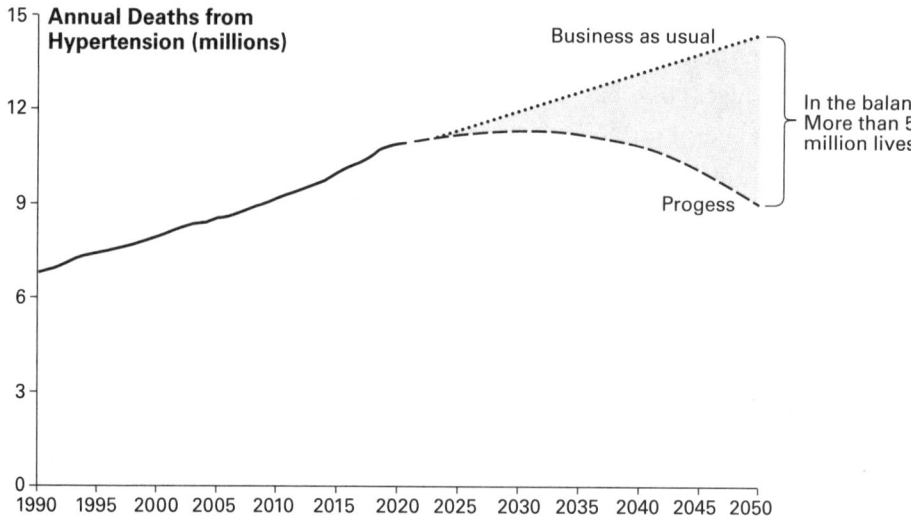

Figure 9.1

Projected hypertension deaths with and without concerted improvement in care. Without urgent action, the number of deaths from hypertension will increase steadily, exceeding 14 million per year by 2050. If there is improved care, the number of deaths will fall to less than 8 million. More than 50 million deaths could be averted by implementing robust blood pressure control interventions. Adapted from Sarah Pickersgill et al., "Modeling Global 80-80-80 Blood Pressure Targets and Cardiovascular Outcomes," *Nature Medicine* 28, no. 8 (July 18, 2022): 1693–1699.

A world without deadly pandemics is within reach. The formula shows how to stop future pandemics and control current ones, including the invisible and deadly pandemic of heart attacks and strokes. This chapter began with a vision of a healthy birth and a long and healthy life. To make that vision become reality, we must apply the formula not only to public health but also to our own lives. To save the most lives, start with the one closest to us—our own.

10   THE FORMULA FOR YOUR HEALTH

Nothing will work unless you do.
—attributed to Maya Angelou

Uncle Dan, my mother's older brother, was the longest-serving law professor in the United States. He retired at age ninety-five and at ninety-eight writes cutting-edge articles on current legal trends. Dan isn't mentally sharp for a ninety-eight-year-old; he's mentally sharp for a thirty-year-old.

It might not seem that the formula for public health progress is relevant to your own health—but it is. The formula to thrive is: See the invisible, including the pathway to progress; believe in the possibility of change; get organized with simplicity to rapidly scale up healthy behaviors. We may not all be as fortunate as Uncle Dan, but by adapting the See/Believe/Create formula, we can maximize the odds that we will live a long, healthy life.

SEE THE FORCES KILLING US

Following the formula, the first step is to see the invisible forces harming us. The question for society is how to save the most lives; the challenge for each of us is to change the things most likely to kill or disable us. As with invisible killers described in chapter 1, we must first see the risks of illnesses, infections, toxins, and trends.

High blood pressure kills more people than any other cause and more than all infectious diseases combined. There's a reason doctors call hypertension the silent killer: The first symptom of high blood pressure is often a heart attack or stroke. Approximately one in three heart attacks is fatal, and many people who survive are disabled. Until 1896, no one had measured blood pressure accurately. Scipione Riva-Rocci, an Italian physician, invented the sphygmomanometer using the inner tube from a bicycle tire, a mercury pressure gauge, and other readily available materials. He made apparent the variation in blood pressure that had been invisible.[1] Elegant epidemiologic studies later proved that every twenty-point increase in the systolic pressure (the first number) starting at 115 doubles the risk of dying from a heart attack or stroke before age seventy.[2] An astonishing two-thirds of people in the United States—and more than 90 percent of people age sixty-five and over—have unhealthy blood pressure.[3] Our unhealthy, salty food and sedentary lives increase blood pressure and also create fatty plaques that block the blood flowing to our heart and brain. This occurs shockingly early in modern lives—by the teenage years.[4]

Tracking progress is also essential for personal health. The New York City community health survey revealed that the smoking decrease had stalled and led us to create new programs that helped hundreds of thousands more New Yorkers quit. Analogously, if we track trends in our own health, we can adjust. Our blood pressure, lipid and blood sugar levels, visual and auditory acuity, and physical fitness can be well within the "normal" range but nevertheless on trajectories toward early disability and death. The "normal" range of each of these is wide and differs among individuals. By knowing and tracking our personal baselines over time, we can make sensible, practical changes to keep them from veering into the abnormal range, by which time far too much damage will have been done. Seeing these risks requires the personal health analog of the public health superpower of surveillance: health care that tracks the otherwise invisible but most important predictors of a long and healthy life, particularly blood pressure, lipid profiles, cancer risk, and other health monitoring.[5] Working with your medical provider to track your numbers and use the information to make real-time improvements through changes in physical activity, food, and medicines can keep these values not only in the "normal" range but in the range that's healthy for you. Genetic and new forms of testing may enable us to see vulnerabilities and risks and tailor treatments and activities to reduce them.[6]

The invisible toxins discussed in chapter 1 also threaten our health. Lead exposure remains a risk, particularly from unregulated cosmetics and spices and from old paint, batteries, and cookware. We can limit exposure to these by making sure regulations are in place and enforced and by avoiding spices and cosmetics that might be contaminated, such as those purchased at unregulated markets. Soot—PM 2.5—is in our air and causes widespread harm but is hard to avoid; HEPA filters can help. We don't know for certain how harmful nanoparticles, microplastics, PFAS and other harmful chemicals are. We can reduce risk by using glass, stainless steel, cast iron, and lead- and PFAS-free ceramics for food preparation and storage; filtering drinking water, if it's contaminated, to remove PFAS and other potentially harmful chemicals; and choosing cosmetics, household items, and clothing made without chemical coatings and certified to be PFAS-free.

The legions of organisms inside each of us—the microbiome—may be our most important and interesting mystery. Microbes are not the enemy. The microbiome consists of trillions of bacteria, viruses, fungi, and archaea, with more than 1,000 different species in your intestines and many more on your skin and mucous membranes. These organisms help with—and in some cases are essential for—digestion, immunity, prevention of allergies, and maybe even mental health.[7] An unhealthy microbiome may be a cause of the obesity epidemic, although our knowledge is still rudimentary.[8] Amazingly, our own intestines are as unexplored as the depths of the ocean or the far side of the moon: Many organisms in our internal microbial forest have yet to be identified. We're just beginning to learn how soap, toothpaste, food, and other exposures affect our microbiome.[9] For a healthy microbiome, it may help to avoid antibiotics except when clearly indicated, eat more fiber and fermented food such as yogurt, limit sugar and processed foods, and get enough sleep and physical activity.[10] As we learn more, we can do more to keep our microbiome and ourselves healthy.

SEE WHAT BLINDS US

To break our personal Cassandra curse, we must recognize and counteract its causes. The same forces that blind society to health threats also cloud personal health decisions. The more we understand what drives our behavior—whether we think of these forces as unconscious motives, ingrained habits, or unrecognized patterns—the better we can change it.

The prevention paradox also applies to personal behaviors: Small changes in physical activity and diet may make no perceptible health difference in the short term but hold the key to a healthier, longer life. Economic factors matter. Healthy food can be more expensive, less accessible, and less convenient. Social norms push us to smoke, drink alcohol, use addictive drugs, and be physically inactive. When we recognize influences on our behavior, we can restructure our environment: find accessible healthy food, identify enjoyable physical activities, and join social networks where healthy behavior is the norm. Understanding that choices are shaped by genes, surroundings, and economic opportunities helps us focus on creating environments that support health rather than blaming ourselves or others for health decisions.[11]

Shortchanging the future, or hyperbolic discounting, results in pursuit of immediate gains and neglect of long-term consequences. It's easier to stay in bed than go for a brisk walk, eat a sweet snack than a healthy one, and skip a routine medical or dental visit. One way to counteract this natural tendency is to make the distant future more vivid. There's an analogy from time management: For years, I accepted invitations to attend work-related events and then regretted having done so. After learning about hyperbolic discounting, I now ask a simple question: If this event were tomorrow, would I go? If not, I decline. Similarly, we can limit the harms of hyperbolic discounting by using logic and emotion to imagine that future health risks and benefits are happening now. More concretely, find healthy behaviors with immediate as well as long-term benefits. Healthy habits are more likely to last if we find physical activities and nutritious foods we love rather than just trying to avoid unhealthy food and sedentary behaviors.

SEE THE PATHWAY TO PROGRESS

With so much controversy about personal health—and so many for-profit ventures that prey on the desire for health—it's tempting to conclude that we simply don't know whether and how to change our behavior. Rigorous analysis can separate sound science from snake oil. Technical rigor, discussed in chapter 3, goes beyond randomized controlled trials to make conclusions, albeit based on imperfect data, that are sufficient to guide behavior. RCTs are fantastic tools, responsible for much of our health progress. Jackhammers are also fantastic tools—but not for fixing your eyeglasses. Technical rigor and the Burden × Amenability formula can help sift through forests of data to show which behaviors matter most and are easiest to improve. This analysis reveals that six factors are the most important to determine whether we live a long and healthy life: blood pressure, lipids, physical activity, nutrition, sleep, and avoidance of substance abuse.

This book does not provide medical advice, and a review of all health interventions is beyond its scope. Advice will change as we learn and will differ for people with different health histories and medical conditions. People who have had a heart attack or stroke require more intensive treatment, as do other high-risk individuals. Your primary health care team remains your source for medical guidance, particularly before starting, changing, or stopping any medical treatment.

Another concept relevant to making decisions about personal health—and one far too rarely acknowledged by the companies and people giving health advice—is the level of certainty that an intervention will improve health. The following three-tier system parallels evidence grading in clinical medicine. In table 10.1, the category "virtually certain" lists interventions with a strong theoretical basis, strong evidence from a wide range of study approaches in multiple countries, and clear demonstration of the effect through intervention trials. There's virtually no possibility of new knowledge changing the conclusion that these actions help. The "strong scientific evidence" category has a theoretical basis, evidence from well-conducted studies, and some evidence of efficacy from ecological or intervention studies. The "some scientific evidence" category has theoretical support and at least one well-conducted study that suggests an effect. A fourth category, not included in table 10.1, includes interventions that are not much more than hunches, with, at present, little or no rigorous supporting evidence despite convincing-sounding theoretical rationales (e.g., paleo diets, fish-oil supplements for everyone, and resveratrol). These and other habits, diets,

Table 10.1

Prioritized list of the most effective ways to live a long and healthy life, stratified by degree of scientific certainty

Virtually certain	Strong scientific evidence	Some scientific evidence
Don't smoke or use other forms of tobacco	Don't vape while continuing to either smoke cigarettes or use other forms of tobacco[12]	Don't vape unless using to quit inhaled tobacco use completely[13]
Keep blood pressure under 120/80[14]		
Control LDL-C cholesterol and ApoB (e.g., to < 80 mg/dL)	Strictly control LDL-C cholesterol and ApoB (e.g., to < 70 mg/dL or lower)[15]	
Be physically active for at least thirty minutes at least four days per week, including improving balance[16]	Improve physical strength and endurance	
Avoid excess alcohol and addictive drugs such as heroin and cocaine	Avoid long-term use of opiates, benzodiazepines, and other psychoactive substances[17]	
Eat a balanced, low-sodium diet with sufficient potassium;[18] don't eat trans fats; avoid sugary beverages and minimize other forms of added sugar	Consume more monounsaturated and polyunsaturated fats; eat plenty of vegetables and fruits; limit consumption of processed meats[19]	Eat a full, healthy breakfast and avoid habitual heavy late meals;[20] reduce red meat consumption;[21] fast intermittently;[22] consume sufficient protein, particularly if vigorously physically active[23]
	Get sufficient (> 7 hours per night) sleep[24]	Get sufficient quality, deep sleep[25]
Get screened for cancer, especially colon, breast, cervical, and skin cancer		
Get recommended vaccines		
Protect and correct hearing and vision; treat depression promptly and fully[26]	Speak a second language or play a musical instrument;[27] avoid traumatic brain injury[28]	Have strong social connections with friends, family, and neighbors;[29] cognitive exercises; B12 supplements even if blood levels are normal;[30] preserve dental and periodontal health[31]

and drugs may extend healthy life, but evidence for their effectiveness remains weak.

One final concept, in addition to Burden × Amenability and level of certainty, is the personal cost-benefit ratio. At one extreme, an intervention that's easy and virtually certain to reduce major health risks (low cost and high amenability) is a no-brainer. Recommended vaccinations are in this category: They can safely and simply prevent some cancers, infections, and painful conditions such as shingles. Other easy and safe interventions may be worthwhile despite uncertain benefit. Oral vitamin B12 supplementation (500–1000 micrograms per day) is in this category. Vitamin B12 measurement, even with the most advanced tests, can miss low levels that impair cognition.[32] Because it's water-soluble, B12 supplementation has essentially no potential harms. For many years, doctors believed that only injections could supplement B12 effectively. Now it's clear that oral supplements, which are much more convenient, can increase levels in most people. Should everyone take B12 supplements? No. Should you? That's up to you. I do—can't hurt, might help, and might even help a lot. And it's cheap. I'd have more confidence in this recommendation if Congress gave the FDA the authority to regulate the quality of nutritional supplements—something the highly profitable supplement industry has blocked for decades. As it is, there's no way to be certain that supplements have the right quantity of the nutrient and don't have harmful contaminants.

Interventions that are difficult and may not have major health benefits are lower priority. Physical endurance training is an example. Few people will be able to do it, although those who do may reap substantial health benefits. I choose healthy foods and physical activities I enjoy rather than try to follow diets or plans I'm unlikely to stick to.

BELIEVE IN OUR HEALTHY FUTURE

Shakespeare wrote of the seven ages of man, ending morosely, "sans teeth, sans eyes, sans taste, sans everything."[33] But these infirmities are not inevitable, dictated by biology. Invisible forces in modern society derail our pathway to healthy aging. Good prevention and care greatly reduce the risk of tooth loss and blindness.[34] People who grow up with ample sunlight are less likely to need corrective lenses.[35] In quieter societies, age-related hearing loss was probably rare.[36] Some preindustrial societies that consumed one-tenth the sodium we consume had no age-related increase in blood pressure.[37] And, most impressively, cognitive super-agers like Uncle Dan don't experience forgetfulness.

Not all preindustrial habits were healthy, nor do people with hypertension, dementia, or loss of teeth, hearing, or vision bring it on themselves. But healthier historical patterns show that each of us, and each of our communities, can be much healthier.

Approaches to break the illusion of inevitability—the *Believe* part of the formula—are relevant in the personal sphere. Appreciating past progress can motivate change and strengthen resolve in the face of challenges and setbacks; people who feel gratitude may have a greater sense of control over their future.[38] Phased improvement is also relevant: Incremental, step-by-step changes in a healthier direction may be more likely to lead to healthy habits.[39] Understanding and celebrating incremental progress and forgiving oneself for lapses in diet and physical activity can help. And, as with rallying the troops for an ambitious public health program, optimism increases motivation. We need to believe that a longer and healthier life is possible: Optimists live longer.[40]

CREATE A HEALTHY FUTURE

It's one thing to see what's killing us and believe we can change; making that change is the biggest challenge. The *create* part of the formula is the hardest for both public and personal health.

Although we don't have unfettered free will, we can improve our health through informed and proactive choices. For both the public and the personal, the first step is to get organized. Our family, friends, work, and social contexts are the personal equivalent of organization. Our environment can increase the likelihood we will make healthier choices. If healthy foods and physical activities are easy, we're more likely to stick with our decisions.

Structural changes help. For example, I put my antihypertensive medications where I can't miss them on my way to get breakfast.

Our health care is another part of our personal health organization. Medical care is complex and problems are often interrelated, so a primary care team is essential. If you're fortunate enough to have access to an integrated system such as Kaiser Permanente, Intermountain Health, Geisinger, or a high-quality primary care clinician, keep it. If possible, find a provider who works as part of a team with nurses, pharmacists, and social workers; medical practices with this model provide better care.[41] For rare or complex conditions, specialists are often essential, but to get the most out of health care—to bridge the gap between scientific knowledge and your health potential—nothing can replace good primary care. In addition to your own clinicians, the most reliable sources of health information are public agencies and some nonprofit organizations such as the Mayo Clinic that look at data rigorously and have limited incentive to recommend for or against any intervention.[42] Clinicians will be able to use newer tools, including genomics, proteomics, and biomarker tests to better see risks and pathways to protection, and newer medications, such as GLP-1 (glucagon-like peptide-1) agonists.

You can improve the six leading drivers of health—blood pressure, lipids, physical activity, nutrition, sleep, and avoidance of substance abuse. Start with hypertension. Beginning in the 1950s, when scientists invented medications to reduce blood pressure, there have been steady improvements in the safety and effectiveness of treatment. By the 1970s, randomized trials proved that medicines for hypertension reduce the risk of stroke, heart failure, heart attack, and death by as much as 75 percent.[43] A blood pressure goal of 120/80 reduces death rates by an additional 27 percent compared to the usual goal of 140/90.[44] The next most powerful way to protect your health is with healthy cholesterol levels. For many people this will mean taking a statin drug and possibly other medications as well. There's controversy about which lipids (different types of fat) in the blood to measure and how low the optimal levels are; LDL-C and ApoB levels below 70 mg/dL are associated with much lower risk of heart attacks and strokes, and even lower levels may be even healthier.[45]

Physical activity is the closest thing to a miracle drug. It reduces cancer, depression, insomnia, dementia, diabetes, hypertension, arthritis, and many other disabling conditions and increases healthy longevity.[46] If you have the personality, resources, and inclination for extensive physical activity, that's great—you'll be much more likely to avoid disability and live independently into old age. I can only stick with activities I enjoy. I play squash, not well but enthusiastically; for the hour I'm on a squash court, that's all I think about, and when I finish, drenched in sweat, endorphins and other beneficial neurochemicals coursing through my body, I can't wait to play again. So, busy as my schedule is, I fit squash in. Try to find vigorous activities you love doing. But if that's not for you, you can still get a large dose of the miracle drug if you build physical activity into your daily routines. This might include taking stairs instead of the elevator, walking farther to work or stores, and bicycling whenever possible. Different types of physical activity work best for different people; a brisk walk, ideally outdoors, is the most accessible. Four brisk walks every week for at least thirty minutes, ideally in a refreshing natural space, can do wonders.[47]

Although controversial and difficult to study accurately, good nutrition is important. There are debates about what healthy nutrition consists of, but you're likely to improve your health if you switch to low-sodium, potassium-enriched salt and use less sodium, eat more vegetables and fruit, limit processed meats, and limit calories, particularly in beverages.[48] "Dieting" usually fails; a better approach is to eat more healthy food you like. Unsalted or lightly salted nuts, vegetables you enjoy, fruits, olive oil, and fish are all healthy and, within reason, the more the better. Foods high in potassium, such as sweet potatoes, salmon, spinach, white beans, avocados, bananas, yogurt, pistachios, tomatoes, and mushrooms tend to be healthy so, again within reason, the more you eat the better.[49] I like sweet red bell peppers, so they're a part of many meals: sliced raw, in salads, roasted, and in cooked dishes. For those who like to count, try calculating the amount of potassium and sodium you consume: The ideal ratio is ≥ 1, that is, at least as much or more potassium than sodium. Nearly everyone now consumes many times more sodium than potassium; flipping this ratio is the strongest dietary predictor of cardiovascular health.[50]

When we eat may also be important. My father, always an astute clinician, noted that many of his obese patients—in an era when obesity was rare—ate little or no breakfast. We metabolize food better when we're active, so the old saying, "Eat breakfast like a king, lunch like a prince, and dinner like a pauper," may have a sound physiological basis. Eating a healthy breakfast and avoiding habitual late and heavy suppers may improve health, although the evidence supporting this is far from definitive.[51]

Sleep has been underrecognized as an important determinant of health and longevity. Adequate sleep appears to preserve memory and problem-solving ability and improves heart, brain, hormonal, and immune functions. Chronic sleep deprivation increases the risk of cardiovascular disease, diabetes, and obesity.[52] Good sleep hygiene can improve sleep quality, although improvement is easier said than done.[53] A regular sleep schedule, a dark and cool bedroom, and avoiding caffeine or nicotine close to bedtime all increase the likelihood of getting a good night's sleep. Managing stress through relaxation techniques and limiting screen exposure before bedtime may enhance sleep duration and quality.[54]

The sixth major determinant of health is avoiding harmful substance use. Tobacco use is the single leading cause of preventable death worldwide (several factors cause hypertension) and damages almost every part of the body. Smoking is responsible for nearly one in six deaths in the United States. Without urgent action, tobacco will kill one billion people globally in this century.[55] Approximately one-third of these deaths are from cardiovascular disease, one-third from cancer, and the rest from respiratory and other diseases. Secondhand smoke increases the risk of heart disease, cancer, and other illnesses in nonsmokers. Smoking doesn't lop off a few unpleasant years at the end of life—it makes unpleasant years a much larger part of much shorter lives. Smokers die about ten years younger than nonsmokers and feel ten years older while alive.[56] It's hard to quit smoking, but the health gain from doing so at any age is enormous; for a smoker, nothing comes close to the health benefit of quitting.[57] Just a few cigarettes or one cigar a day drastically increase the risk of a heart attack.[58] Sadly, this basic fact can be obscured by the latest fads and scares. Most Americans who have ever smoked have already quit, and nicotine patches, gum, and other medications at least double the likelihood of success. People who smoke when they wake up, smoke half a pack of cigarettes a day or more, or struggle to avoid smoking in nonsmoking places are heavily addicted and much more likely to quit if they receive multiple medications and comprehensive support.

Alcohol causes health harms including cancer and damage to the heart, brain, liver, and peripheral nerves. It worsens depression and increases violence and social disruption.[59] The purported finding that small amounts of alcohol are healthy, heavily promoted by the alcohol industry, resulted from the classic error of J-shaped curve interpretation discussed in chapter 3. Analyzed accurately, the health risks of alcohol are linear: The more you drink, the less healthy it is, and there is no health benefit from drinking small quantities. This doesn't mean you shouldn't drink any alcohol. As with other behaviors, a risk/benefit calculation—at least an informal one!—can guide your decisions. If having one or two drinks at a special time is important to you, you can certainly choose to do so; most people will have minimal or no negative health impacts from this level of consumption. More serious problems come with binge drinking, underage drinking, regular heavy drinking, drinking while pregnant, and drinking and driving.[60] Beginning to drink before adulthood impairs cognitive development and increases the risk of lifelong unhealthy drinking patterns.

The epidemic of opiate addiction in the United States has lasted for a quarter of a century and killed more than a million people. The initial catalyst of this tragedy was pharmaceutical companies' fraudulent and aggressive marketing, which led to massive overprescription of opiate medications.[61] Opiates are an important part of modern medical care for short-term (i.e., three days or less) very severe pain, but have little or no role in treatment of chronic pain because they reduce the likelihood of recovery and increase the risk of death.[62] They are highly addictive. Their use reflects poor management of both pain and addiction in the US health care system. Similarly, doctors prescribe benzodiazepines such as Xanax and Valium for insomnia, anxiety, and other conditions, but these medications are also addictive, increase the risk of falls and memory loss, and can exacerbate depression. Short-term use or use when managed by a psychiatrist as part of mental health care may be beneficial, but the vast majority of prescriptions for benzodiazepines are unnecessary or harmful.[63] The same is true of amphetamines such as Adderall and Dexedrine, except when used as part of a comprehensive program to treat attention-deficit disorder, a condition that is greatly overdiagnosed, or for the rare condition of narcolepsy.[64]

These prescription patterns reflect an unfortunate reality: We overmedicate conditions that have symptoms and undermedicate conditions that don't. Medicines for pain, anxiety, and hyperactivity are overprescribed and overused; medications for silent conditions such as high blood pressure, high cholesterol, and hepatitis C infection are underprescribed and underused. The most visible conditions are rarely the most lethal—harms that are invisible kill many more people.

The health effects of marijuana use remain controversial. Marijuana can reduce nausea and improve appetite for people with cancer and reduce pain and discomfort for people with multiple sclerosis. Marijuana can exacerbate mental illness, increase motor vehicle crashes, and cause problems in infants whose mothers used it during pregnancy. Long-term use is associated with lung problems.[65] It can be addictive and may decrease effective functioning, particularly for people who begin using it at a younger age.[66]

Each of the six healthy habits—controlling blood pressure, reducing unhealthy lipids, being physically active, eating healthy, sleeping well, and avoiding harmful substance use—increases our chance of living the life we choose for longer. Simple changes increase the odds we will adopt healthy behaviors.[67] Interactions among these habits create powerful synergies. For example, controlling blood pressure increases the odds that we can continue regular physical activity, and regular physical activity reduces blood pressure. A healthy diet and sufficient sleep reduce blood pressure. Avoiding excess alcohol use reduces blood pressure and decreases the risk of injury and cognitive decline. And prevention of cognitive decline may be the single most important element of healthy longevity.

PREVENT DEMENTIA

My beloved grandmother Evelyn, a widow from her fifties, lived independently into her nineties. She and I were close, and I often visited her to chat (and eat the cookies and chocolate she always had around in abundance). Once when I stopped by, she was flipping her mattress—at age ninety. Startled, I asked why she was doing this. "Oh," she said, "I was told that if you do this every week, the mattress lasts longer." The only thing she feared was dementia. At every visit, she clutched my arm tightly and shared her terror that she would lose her prodigious memory (able to recite long passages of Shakespeare and romantic poetry from memory into her nineties) and live out her days, undignified, in a nursing home. She pleaded with me to prevent this, but, sadly, it's exactly what happened. She spent the last years of her life unaware of her surroundings, in a nursing home, biting at and fighting with nursing staff, unable to communicate. I felt I had failed her. (My father, who saw this tragedy unfold, requested that if he were admitted to a nursing home, I report that he was allergic to nutritional supplements—the milkshake-like drinks that sustained my grandmother for those last miserable years.) Of all infirmities, loss of cognitive faculties most undermines our humanity. Short of euthanasia, how could Evelyn have avoided the ending she so dreaded? Most of the measures are the six keys discussed above, with some additions and nuances.

We can increase our odds of being a cognitive super-ager—Uncle Dan, not Grandmother Evelyn (although being able to quote Shakespeare at length at age ninety isn't bad). Some super-agers are simply lucky—despite unhealthy behaviors, factors we don't understand allow them to escape memory loss and other disabilities. But even if you haven't won the longevity lottery, you can still make choices that promote healthy aging.

Table 10.1 and appendix 2 show healthy behaviors, including the six key habits discussed above, that increase our odds of living a long, healthy, and dementia-free life. Avoiding tobacco and limiting alcohol consumption prevent memory loss. Controlling blood pressure, ideally to 120/80 or below, reduces the risk of stroke and dementia.[68] Prevention or correction of vision and hearing loss, avoidance of traumatic brain injury, and prompt treatment of depression all reduce the risk of dementia.[69] Regular physical activity is likely to reduce this risk.[70] People with stronger social networks—strong connections with family, friends, and neighbors—may live longer and healthier, with less dementia.[71]

Measures beyond these steps are either less certain to reduce dementia or harder to implement. Having more education correlates with a longer, more independent life.[72] Speaking at least two languages fluently or playing a musical instrument reduces the risk of Alzheimer's disease.[73] Consistent intellectual challenges may preserve mental capacity.[74] Certain medications for diabetes, medications to reduce cholesterol, and GLP-1 receptor agonists may have substantial cognitive and other health benefits.[75] Less exposure to air pollution may reduce risk.[76] There is some evidence that vaccination against herpes zoster virus (shingles) reduces the risk of dementia.[77] Perhaps the most controversial area is whether healthy eating reduces the risk of cognitive decline. Although miracle, mind-preserving diets don't exist, healthy eating for decades is likely to reduce the risk of dementia, not least from reducing blood pressure and the risk of stroke.[78]

PERSONAL POLITICS

Our environment shapes our choices. Today only 3 percent of adults in the United States have the four most important basic healthy habits: not smoking, regular physical activity, eating at least five servings of vegetables and fruits a day, and being at a healthy weight. In other words, the odds of having these four habits are more than 30:1 against us.[79] Advocating for healthy policies is in our self-interest. With healthy policies, it's more likely that children reach adulthood free from addiction to tobacco, alcohol, and other drugs; with healthy social and emotional development; with healthy habits of eating, physical activity, sleep, and electronics use; and at a healthy weight. Despite the best parenting, less than 5 percent of children will have these healthy outcomes. We can make this future the norm if we use the lightning Mark Twain described and Mike Bloomberg has led: policy change to make healthy choices the default choices.

We can increase physical activity by joining with others to advocate for streets that make it easier for people to walk and bicycle; this can improve both health and the local economy. At the state level, increasing taxes on tobacco, alcohol, sugary drinks and other unhealthy foods will reduce use of these products, especially by kids. Nationally, advocacy for comprehensive primary health care could transform our current disease-care system into a true health care system that adequately funds primary health care and holds it accountable for preventing disability and disease. Advocating for broader changes isn't just the right thing to do—it could save our lives.

The formula shows the pathway to a healthier, more resilient future.

EPILOGUE: A HEALTHY WORLD

In 1997, leading Indian physicians opposed the new tuberculosis control program; I invited Sir John Crofton to address a consensus conference. Knighted for discovering how to cure tuberculosis, Crofton—then in his late eighties—hadn't lost a bit of his intelligence, strategic thinking, or humility. Along with American tuberculosis expert Dr. John Sbarbaro, he helped convince Indian academic physicians to endorse the program.

At the end of the fruitful visit, I invited Sir John to my home in New Delhi. A large new loan from the World Bank would fund expansion of effective tuberculosis control services to much of the country. Projects using Karel Styblo's approach were beginning to perform well. It was a pleasant, sunny afternoon. I commented that, with technological advances and headway on health and other social programs, it seemed that global progress is inevitable.

The moment I said that, it was as if a shadow had fallen across the room. Sir John became deadly serious. His usual twinkling cheerfulness evaporated. Tears came to his eyes. "During World War II, I served in the British Army as a doctor. I retreated across Africa and across Europe as we lost one battle after another. If FDR hadn't gotten the Americans into the war when he did, Hitler would have won. Progress is *not* inevitable."

Problems ranging from climate change to antimicrobial resistance to drug addiction show that progress requires sustained effort. For some issues, public health advocates must work for decades, as they did to reduce drunk driving.[1] Despite substantial progress, deaths from tuberculosis in India remain common.[2]

Optimism may seem naïve, but it's grounded in reality. Many harms—such as those from oil spills, lead poisoning, and air pollution—are decreasing, while agricultural yields, literacy, female education, and other healthy trends continue to increase.[3] Sir John often encouraged others with the comment that we're going from strength to strength, success to success. Phased progress makes substantial further progress possible.

Clean water, sanitary food, and better living conditions reduced infections and extended healthy life expectancy in the twentieth century. Today, the tobacco, alcohol, junk food, gun, and fossil fuel industries are the deadliest vectors of disease. They work to negate each part of the formula: They obscure their products' harms and undermine science so that it's harder to see the damage their products cause and the way forward; they erode belief in progress; and they block public health action. One false narrative these industries promote is that public health is a barrier to economic progress. In fact, better health—including through reduction of the harms these industries cause—accelerates economic progress.[4] Adam Smith, who provided the conceptual underpinning of modern capitalism 250 years ago, recognized that tobacco, alcohol, and sugar are "nowhere necessaries of life" and are therefore "extremely proper subjects of taxation."[5]

We can see the harms killer industries cause, believe in the possibility of further progress, and create a healthier future. To overcome industry opposition and save lives, we must tax tobacco, alcohol, sugary and salty foods, and carbon; reduce air pollution; structure communities to encourage walking and bicycling; make healthy foods more accessible and affordable than unhealthy foods; and create effective, accountable primary health care systems.

Improving primary health care is particularly important because the potential health gains from clinical medicine are increasing. From tuberculosis (the former leading killer) to hypertension (today's leading killer) to many cancers, chronic diseases, and HIV, treatment can protect and restore health. Unfortunately, doctors in the US gave patients the right care only about half the time and harmful care nearly a fifth of the time.[6] Lack of effective primary health care creates a chasm between the miracles of modern medicine and the millions of lives these miracles could save.

The formula shows how to close the primary care gap (see appendix 1 for ready-reference guide). *See* what's invisible: 100 million people in the US and most people around the world lack a primary care provider, increasing health care costs and causing avoidable suffering and death. See the forces that blind us to the drivers of this unhealthy pattern. And see the path forward—the technical package for primary health care described in chapter 3. Recognize and overcome economic and political opposition so the overarching incentives of the health care system begin to strengthen primary care. Make visible the performance of the system, especially for the groups most in need and conditions that can improve health the most. Select a small number of indicators, ensure they're accurate, and work with doctors, nurses, pharmacists, outreach workers, and patients to improve them. Are strokes, heart attacks, and the hospitalizations they require being prevented? What proportion of people with hypertension have it under control? What proportion of people with an indication for a statin are receiving one? What proportion of women receive the contraceptive method that meets their needs and preferences? What proportion of children get vaccinated on schedule?

Believe we can make progress by recognizing past achievements, building on successes, and cultivating optimism. Experience in countries as varied as Costa Rica, the United Kingdom, and Thailand suggests that as primary health care improves, a virtuous cycle can begin. Better care leads patients and communities to appreciate primary care more. Politicians then take note and further increase funding. As the cycle continues, primary care can escape partisan politics and become a national commitment. The vicious cycle of more and more specialty care can change to a virtuous cycle of more and better primary health care and healthier people.[7]

The playbook for political progress outlined in chapter 8 shows how to *create* better primary care: Identify who wins and who loses if the system changes and implement the winning triad—strong government, vibrant civil society, and accurate, real-time monitoring. Internal government reform teams can lead efforts, and, although progress is usually slow and incremental, advocates can accelerate change.[8] Each community and health care system can choose the conditions to focus on—the ones that harm the most people and are most amenable to progress. When health care systems track these outcomes and tie payments to improvement, the value of our health care system—and the number of lives saved—will increase rapidly.

The See/Believe/Create formula can also help tackle broader challenges such as climate change. We increasingly see its current and future harms. Hurricanes and heat waves lead the news, but subtler impacts could be deadlier. Environmental changes increase population migration and conflict. Warmer environments increase the spread of malaria, dengue, Lyme disease, cholera, and other diseases. Food and water insecurity is increasing, and with these, drought and crop failures. Air pollution from wildfires and fossil fuels increases lung and heart disease.[9] But there are good reasons to believe a sustainable future is within reach. In the past decade, renewable energy prices have plummeted, with solar panels now 90 percent and wind turbines approximately 40 percent cheaper.[10] In many parts of the world, renewable energy is now less expensive than fossil fuel. Electric vehicles accelerate the transition to a low-carbon economy.[11] There's precedent for progress: The ozone layer is recovering, thanks to a global agreement reached when the world heeded the Cassandra warning and avoided catastrophe.[12]

Phased transition to cleaner energy sources is underway. Today, the United Kingdom burns less coal than at any time since 1662, when John Graunt published his groundbreaking analysis of mortality—and hypothesized that coal smoke increased death rates. Since 2010, the Beyond Coal campaign, backed by the Sierra Club and funded by Bloomberg Philanthropies, has begun closing more than two-thirds of the coal plants in the United States.[13] This reduces greenhouse gas emissions and saves billions of dollars in health care costs every year. Technological advances may make carbon capture safe and feasible at scale. For the Create component, organization, scalable solutions, and effective communication will be essential, but progress depends on the political approach outlined in chapter 8. To succeed, we must identify winners and losers, deciders and influencers; support governmental institutions committed to change; increase advocacy; and ensure rigorous monitoring and accountability. Although decades of accumulating emissions and environmental feedback loops make climate change increasingly difficult to slow or reverse, these steps can make country and global action more effective.

The formula can also accelerate progress on other societal priorities. We can expose the often-invisible inefficiencies and inequities in current transportation systems, break the illusion that these are insurmountable, and create better systems through technical innovation, operational excellence, and political savvy. Better public transportation increases economic opportunities, reduces pollution and climate change, and promotes physical activity. Successful models, including integrated transit networks in Copenhagen and Seoul, demonstrate that public transportation can be reliable and inclusive.

Education promotes health and is a cornerstone of societal progress. To improve it, we must see the health and societal costs of ineffective schools and establish the pathways to progress. Finland's education reforms and online platforms such as Khan Academy show that improvements are possible. Success requires that we expose disparities, challenge the misconception that these gaps are unchangeable, increase and align resources to address children's needs in and out of the classroom, and use data to improve student and teacher performance.

This book doesn't attempt to address every important health problem, nor is the formula the only route to improvement. The most effective efforts track outcomes systematically and change course in real time to accelerate progress. Similarly, more evidence and experience can undoubtedly improve the See/Believe/Create formula and the specific actions needed to implement it.

In the preface, I predicted that the pandemic of heart attacks and strokes—today's leading cause of death—will end in the coming decades. The formula shows how. See silent killers such as hypertension, unhealthy lipid levels, and air pollution. Believe we can end these pandemics as we ended earlier pandemics of smallpox, diphtheria, and tetanus. Counteract the forces that increase tobacco use, unhealthy diets, and air pollution. Because our health depends on our community's policies and programs, build coalitions to create a healthier future. Well-organized, prioritized actions that manage the political and economic drivers of ill health make success possible.

For the past four decades, I've tried to use empiricism to learn what's killing people, partner with others to save lives, and confront brutally honest data about program failure and success. I'm optimistic. Public health has saved billions of lives. Sir John was right that progress isn't inevitable, but our world is healthier, more connected, and has better tools and more knowledge than ever in human history. When we as a society work together to implement the formula—to reveal then overcome the forces and illnesses that block our paths—millions of people, including you and your family, will enjoy longer, healthier lives.

Acknowledgments

This book results from ten years of writing and forty years of work in public health.

Patients, advocates, and many mentors have taught me. The study in Douglas, Tennessee, was a project of the Appalachian Student Health Coalition, part of the Center for Health Services at Vanderbilt University. Richard Couto and Barbara Clinton led that program, and the job formed my perspective and understanding of health. Eleanor Bell, my supervisor when I was an Epidemic Intelligence Service Officer, showed the importance of attention to detail, technical knowledge, and deep caring. Dr. Kelly Henning, another supervisor during my EIS training, has remained a friend and colleague in the thirty-five years since, demonstrating repeatedly what Aristotle described as practical wisdom or, more simply, the best judgment of anyone I've ever worked with. Staff of the CDC helped me learn as an EIS officer and later as I became a tuberculosis specialist. Louis Salinas was my coach, critic, and partner in public health for thirty years, including leading my transition to the role of CDC director. I have succeeded in public health to the extent I learned from Louis and failed when I didn't.

Tuberculosis control specialists are a unique society of siblings. At one point, three of my tuberculosis mentors had a combined 200 years working in the field: Dr. Bill Harris, the wonderful medical director of the New York City tuberculosis program, who, despite being in his eighties and increasingly disabled, drove to every health department clinic to meticulously review every medical record; George Comstock (chapter 3); and Sir John

Crofton (epilogue). I'm deeply grateful to have had the opportunity to learn from them and from Dr. Karel Styblo, who appears throughout this book. During my time in India, I learned from the wonderful Dr. Fabio Luelmo and the indomitable Dr. G. R. Khatri as well as from an unsung, remarkable physician, Dr. T. Santha Devi. Dr. Devi, I believe, understood tuberculosis treatment better than anyone in the world. She participated in or analyzed every important tuberculosis trial and bridged the understanding of a great clinician with the analytic skills of a great researcher. Dr. Devi's mastery of these issues informed my understanding of the strengths and limitations of randomized controlled trials.

Being health commissioner under Mayor Mike Bloomberg was the greatest stroke of luck of my career. Bloomberg challenged us to be creative and fearless, demonstrated how to manage and delegate effectively, and has the unique combination of outsized success in business, politics, and philanthropy. Hundreds of thousands of people in New York City and tens of millions of people around the world are living longer and healthier lives because of Bloomberg's strategic leadership. The team at the New York City Health Department showed what a great public health agency can achieve when it combines rigorous science with effective implementation and is backed by a political leader like Mike Bloomberg whose most basic value is to do the right thing.

As New York City health commissioner and then director of the CDC, I had the privilege of learning from hundreds of doctors, veterinarians, dentists, and other public health specialists, too numerous to name, who dedicate their careers to public health. They are unsung heroes, protecting and improving lives through the usually invisible work of building knowledge, tracking trends, and implementing and improving programs.

Bill Foege has been a mentor and friend for more than thirty years. In late-night calls to his home in Seattle from mosquito-infested phone booths in rural India, Bill guided and encouraged me. Bill also suggested the concept that public health surveillance reveals a world otherwise as invisible as the microscopic world.

Staff of Resolve to Save Lives helped refine many of the concepts in this book. Amanda McClelland shows how essential it is to listen to and understand communities and suggested the risk-alert level framework to modulate COVID restrictions. Erin Sykes provided a thoughtful perspective and useful suggestions on public health communication. Marine Buisson-niére greatly improved the analysis of the political aspects of public health and, with her encyclopedic knowledge, provided examples of effective non-governmental organizations.

Two people read many versions of this book. Richard Garfield has been a friend and colleague for more than forty years. Richard's insights strengthened description of the practical aspects of public health, spared readers tedious detail, and greatly improved the book. Family, friends, and colleagues were generous with their time and made this work stronger and more rigorous: Charles Barber, Karen Brudney, Shama Cash-Goldwasser, Jesse Chang-Frieden, Michael Chang-Frieden, Antonio Dajer, Jenab Diallo, Richard Doner, Thomas Farley, Carl Frieden, Jeffry Frieden, Ken Frieden, Sari Frieden, Denri Gottemaker, Kelly Henning, Corby Kummer, Jessica Leighton, Barron Lerner, Elizabeth Kolbert, Cyrus Shahpar, and Eric Topol. Dr. James Pirkle provided feedback and references for the section on tobacco and nicotine. Dr. Edwin Mitchell reviewed and provided important input to the section describing the work he and others did to document the major cause and prevention of sudden infant death. Dr. Stuart Nichol clarified the Marburg and Ebola incidents. Drew Blakeman assisted with essays and scientific articles that are precursors of the book. All errors are, of course, solely my responsibility.

Thanks to MIT Press editorial director Janice Audet for superb input ranging from the title to the structure to the organization, content, and style of chapters. Without her collaboration, many concepts of this book would have been lost in a blizzard of unnecessary complexity. Thanks also to James Levine, my agent, for believing in the book, for persisting, and for his support. Andrew Wylie provided wise guidance on earlier versions of this project; the reader will determine how well I've adhered to one of Andrew's many wonderful dicta—to cut out the parts people would skip.

Rochelle Sun provided outstanding research assistance. Her meticulous work was instrumental to document and improve the book. We selected references to credit originators of ideas, present up-to-date data, and provide thorough reviews. We have not referenced other relevant articles due to constraints of space. Quotations without citations are from conversations. I used the large language model ChatGPT as a thesaurus, grammar checker, and virtual research assistant and the Claude model to discuss stylistic improvements. In all cases, I verified the information provided.

My family has made my work and this book possible. Work has taken me away from family more than I wish to remember, and I thank them for their understanding. My mother, Professor Nancy Frieden, is editor-in-chief of our clan. Her willingness to read multiple drafts of the entire manuscript and provide line edits and thoughtful feedback made the book much more readable.

Finally, I am deeply indebted to the patients, doctors, nurses, pharmacists, outreach workers, and other health care workers who have taught me so much. Being a doctor is a privilege; every patient is a universe, bringing unique perspectives. Being a public health doctor for entire communities intensifies that privilege. The experiences and resilience of patients, health staff, and communities inspired and shaped this book and also me and my work. Words cannot convey my gratitude.

Ready-Reference Guide for Community-Wide Action

The formula is first to see what may not be readily visible:

- Microbes, toxins, and trends that can harm people.
- The status of programs to address these harms.
- The pathway to progress, based on a rigorous understanding of all forms of evidence, including practical experience from attempts to implement programs.

The second part of the formula is to believe in the possibility of change:

- Recognize past progress.
- Make step-by-step, phase-wise progress in at least two different areas with good leadership and careful support, learning and optimizing the approach in the early phases.
- Cultivate and maintain optimism while avoiding the optimism bias and misguided optimism.

The third part of the formula is to create:

- Organize systematically and address large problems by breaking them into manageable sections.
- Prioritize important but nonurgent initiatives.
- Improve teams and organizations in both public and private sectors through better hiring, transparency, and a focus on mission, pragmatism, and use of data to improve performance.

- Use simplicity to facilitate speed and scale and reach entire populations.
- Communicate effectively by listening well and creating the right message, delivered by the right messenger to the right audience at the right time to build trust and counter misinformation.
- Make political progress by identifying and organizing winners and losers, deciders and influencers, advocates and partners, and by mitigating commercial interests, getting funding, and strengthening government's appropriate role promoting and protecting health. Pragmatism and timing are essential to success.

Table A1.1

Forces that drive the Cassandra curse and mitigation strategies

Driver	Mitigation
Prevention paradox (small individual changes lead to large societal changes) and the economic and political corollary of concentrated costs and diffuse benefits	• Increase awareness of collective benefits • Appeal to community cohesiveness and responsibility to children and future generations • Align incentives by providing short-term benefits or subsidies to compensate direct costs • Regulate to reduce harms
Economic forces	• Uncover hidden economic interests • Harness aligned interests • Build coalitions to overcome self-interested entities that work against health • Find funding for programs that promote health
The myth of unfettered free will	• Reveal and counteract forces that undermine free choice
False alarms	• Prepare people for the inevitability of false alarms • Increase the proportion of alarms that are accurate
Institutional, cultural, and social norms	• Identify community leaders, media strategies, and healthy cultural norms to counteract unhealthy norms • Show that current norms are neither normal nor inevitable and that the norm was absent or different in the past • Recognize that patience may be required while impatiently working for change
Hyperbolic discounting (shortchanging the future)	• Make the future visible with models, vivid personal stories, descriptions of future reality, and imagining that the distant future is tomorrow • Compensate for the distance of future benefits with immediate benefits

Table A1.2

Examples of tips to see the invisible, believe in the possibility of progress, and create a healthier future

Action	Tips
See the invisible	• Invest in and improve tracking systems • Investigate current actual and potential silent harms • Use predictive analytics to make likely future scenarios visible
Believe: Shatter the illusion of inevitability	• Show past progress • Make phased progress • Innovate • Cultivate optimism and a sense of control in individuals, organizations, and communities
Create a healthier future through technical rigor, operational excellence, and political power	
Technical rigor	• Analyze scientific findings and practical realities carefully, incorporating an understanding of strengths and weaknesses of all data inputs and the value of practice-based evidence • Create a culture of continuous improvement and transparency based on the best available evidence • Bridge the learning-versus-doing divide • Use the Burden × Amenability formula to identify programs and approaches most likely to have a large health benefit • Make progress on as basic a level of the public health impact pyramid (figure 3.1) as possible • Establish focused technical packages most likely to result in progress • Stay humble
Operational excellence	• Organize, including through incident management systems in all emergencies • Use a four-quadrant framework (table 5.1) to prioritize actions that maximize impact and efficiency • Get hiring, procurement, management, and communication right • Use simplicity and speed to achieve scale • Strengthen institutions by improving political and organizational alignment, management, and technical skills and by managing risks, strengthening leadership, and planning for sustainability • Ensure clarity of mission, connection with front-line realities, and real-time, accurate information systems to track and improve program performance
Political power	• Find and fight winnable battles • Identify winners and losers, deciders and influencers, advocates and partnerships • Be pragmatic and identify windows of opportunity • Support champions and teams within government • Support individuals and groups outside of government to advocate for and support societal progress • Identify and mitigate opposition to health-promoting actions • Create and foster partnerships • Establish rigorous, transparent, accurate public tracking • Get sufficient funds

Ready-Reference Guide: Proven Steps to a Long, Healthy Life

WARNING: Most health advice in the media and on the internet is driven by profit, hype, or sloppy thinking.

The table below outlines proven (•••) likely (••), and possible (•) ways to live a long, disability-free life. The table lists actions in descending order of impact and indicates the level of certainty of each.

High blood pressure kills more people than any other cause. The first symptom is often a heart attack or stroke. Every 20-point increase in systolic blood pressure starting at 115 doubles your risk of heart attack or stroke; aim for a blood pressure of <120/80. Two thirds of Americans and more than 90 percent of those over sixty-five have unhealthy blood pressure. High blood pressure is the "silent killer"—it causes damage with every heartbeat.

High levels of unhealthy *cholesterol and other lipids* damage arteries, leading to heart attacks, strokes and other disabilities. Fatty plaques block blood flow to the heart and brain, with damage starting by the teenage years. The lower the levels, the lower the risk.

Tobacco, alcohol, and other toxic substances shorten lives and increase disability. Tobacco remains the world's leading preventable cause of death. Smokers die about ten years younger than nonsmokers and feel a decade older while alive. Alcohol increases cancer risk, damages heart, brain, liver, and nerves, and causes a wide range of harms. Other toxins, including lead, PM 2.5 (soot), and "forever chemicals," can silently harm health.

Physical activity is the closest thing to a miracle drug. Whatever a person's weight, physical activity reduces the risk of cancer, heart disease, diabetes, depression, arthritis, dementia, and many other conditions. Regular activity improves heart, brain, strength, bones, balance, mental health, and cognitive function.

Food choices can improve blood pressure, cholesterol, weight, and help determine how well and how long we live. What we eat affects our microbiome, inflammation, and disease risk.

Adequate sleep is crucial for physical health, cognitive function, and emotional wellbeing. During sleep, our body repairs damage, consolidates memories, and maintains immune function. Insufficient or poor quality sleep increases the risk of obesity, diabetes, cardiovascular disease, depression, and dementia.

The following table uses the best available evidence to estimate the impact of actions that increase longevity and prevent dementia.[1] See note 1 for methods and caveats. Having a good primary health care team makes many of these actions more achievable.

Table A2.1

Action	Approximate healthy life expectancy gain (months)	Strength of evidence for longevity benefit	Strength of evidence for dementia prevention	Tip
Don't use tobacco, and if you do, quit[2]	120	•••	•••	Use cessation medicines, which double quit success
Keep blood pressure under 120/80[3]	36–48	•••	•••	Take medicines daily and check blood pressure regularly
Control unhealthy lipids (LDL-C and ApoB)[4]	24–36	•••	•••	Statins and other medications work well
Exercise for at least 30 minutes at least 4 days/week[5]	24–36	•••	•••	Find physical activity you enjoy; add balance exercises if you're older
Average no more than 1 alcoholic drink/day for women and 2 drinks/day for men[6]	24	•••	•••	Find alternative drinks and contexts you enjoy; avoid binge drinking (>4 drinks for men and >3 for women)
Eat a low-sodium diet with sufficient potassium[7]	12–18	•••	••	Eat high-potassium foods such as sweet potato, salmon, spinach, white beans, avocado, bananas, yogurt, pistachios, tomatoes, and mushrooms; switch to potassium-enriched low-sodium salt; eat more potassium than sodium
Protect and correct vision and hearing[8]	12–18	•	••	Get regular check-ups and follow up; avoid loud noises, if hearing is impaired, correct early and use aids regularly to reduce cognitive decline
Have strong social connections[9]	6–18	•	••	Find friends who listen to you and who you enjoy listening to
Replace unhealthy with healthy fats[10]	6–12	••	•	Replace unhealthy fats with monounsaturated (e.g. olive oil, nuts) and polyunsaturated fats (e.g. fish, soy)
Avoid processed meats[11]	6–12	••	•	Find healthy foods you enjoy, especially plant-based meals

Action	Approximate healthy life expectancy gain (months)	Strength of evidence for longevity benefit	Strength of evidence for dementia prevention	Tip
Avoid sugary beverages[12]	6–12	•	•	Water is the healthiest beverage and coffee and tea (ideally without sugar) are fine; sugary drinks, including fruit juices, are mostly empty calories
Get at least 7 hours of sleep with good sleep quality[13]	4–8	•	•	Keep a consistent sleep schedule and cool and dark bedroom; avoid caffeine, nicotine, alcohol and digital device use close to bedtime
Get recommended cancer screenings and follow-up[14]	4	••	No evidence	Colon cancer screening is particularly important
Use HEPA filters[15]	0–2	•	•	Use and regularly replace HEPA filters if you live in a polluted area
Get recommended vaccines[16]	Substantial; the amount depends on infection risk	•••	•	Stay on schedule to protect yourself and your family
Avoid brain injury[17]	Brain injury may shorten life expectancy substantially	•••	•••	Bicycle helmets (especially for kids); road safety (especially for young adults); fall prevention (especially for older adults)
Treat depression[18]	Likely but not well documented	•	••	Get professional help: medications and therapy can be effective
Speak a second language and/ or play a musical instrument[19]	Not documented to extend life	Limited or no evidence	••	Use a second language in conversation or play a musical instrument regularly to increase cognitive reserve

Proven (•••) likely (••), and possible (•) ways to live a longer, dementia-free life.

Notes

PREFACE

1. Karen Brudney and Jay F. Dobkin, "Resurgent Tuberculosis in New York City: Human Immunodeficiency Virus, Homelessness, and the Decline of Tuberculosis Control Programs," *American Review of Respiratory Disease* 144, no. 4 (October 1, 1991): 745–749.

2. Michael D. Iseman, "Treatment of Multidrug-Resistant Tuberculosis," *New England Journal of Medicine* 329, no. 11 (September 9, 1993): 784–791; Thomas R. Frieden et al., "A Multi-Institutional Outbreak of Highly Drug-Resistant Tuberculosis," *JAMA* 276, no. 15 (October 16, 1996): 1229–1235.

3. C.-E. A. Winslow, *The Life of Hermann M. Biggs, M.D., D. Sc., LL. D., Physician and Statesman of the Public Health* (Pennsylvania: Lea & Febiger, 1929), 143–144.

4. Thomas R. Frieden et al., "The Emergence of Drug-Resistant Tuberculosis in New York City," *New England Journal of Medicine* 328 (February 25, 1993): 521–526.

5. Bolajoko O. Olusanya et al., "Developmental Disabilities Among Children Younger Than 5 Years in 195 Countries and Territories, 1990–2016: A Systematic Analysis for the Global Burden of Disease Study 2016," *Lancet Global Health* 6, no. 10 (October 1, 2018): e1100–1121.

6. Thomas McKeown, *The Role of Medicine: Dream, Mirage, or Nemesis?* (Oxford: Blackwell, 1979), xvi, 207.

CHAPTER 1

1. R. L. Riley et al., "Aerial Dissemination of Pulmonary Tuberculosis: A Two-Year Study of Contagion in a Tuberculosis Ward," *American Journal of Epidemiology* 70, no. 2 (September 1, 1959): 185–196. Viruses known as bacteriophages (literally, organisms that eat bacteria) infect bacteria. Analysis of bacteriophage patterns of different tuberculosis strains provided an early, albeit imprecise, way to see trends inside of microbes.

2. Thomas R. Frieden et al., "The Molecular Epidemiology of Tuberculosis in New York City: The Importance of Nosocomial Transmission and Laboratory Error," *Tubercle and Lung*

Disease 77, no. 5 (October 1, 1996): 407–413. In the following decades, genomic finger-printing technology continued to improve. By the time COVID hit in 2020, it was possible to track the spread of subgroups of the virus, known as clades, as they spread around the world. Remarkably, a single mutation in just one of the 30,000 RNA bases that instruct the virus how to develop caused a substantial increase in infectivity, resulting in explosive spread.

3.   Frieden et al., "A Multi-Institutional Outbreak of Highly Drug-Resistant Tuberculosis."

4.   Martin I. Meltzer et al., "Estimating the Future Number of Cases in the Ebola Epidemic—Liberia and Sierra Leone, 2014–2015," *Morbidity and Mortality Weekly Report, Supplement* 63, no. 03 (September 26, 2014). There has been criticism of Meltzer's model, for example because it assumes that no improvement in control measures would be implemented in the following months despite the increase in cases. Meltzer's fundamental observation remains valid: Cases were increasing exponentially and would continue to do so until effective control measures were implemented. Ron Klain, the White House Ebola coordinator, quipped that if you took a left turn instead of a right turn after driving over the George Washington Bridge from New York to New Jersey, you'd realize you weren't going north before you arrived in Florida. The model projected accurately what would happen if there were no improvement in the disease control activities. When public health efforts succeed and control an outbreak, it may appear that the response was an overreaction. For criticism of Meltzer's model, see Gerardo Chowell et al., "Perspectives on Model Forecasts of the 2014–2015 Ebola Epidemic in West Africa: Lessons and the Way Forward," *BMC Medicine* 15, no. 1 (March 1, 2017). For comparison of Meltzer's model to other Ebola models, see Cécile Viboud et al., "The RAPIDD Ebola Forecasting Challenge: Synthesis and Lessons Learnt," *Epidemics* 22 (March 2018): 13–21. For a detailed evaluation of Meltzer's model, see Robert Gaffey and Cécile Viboud, "Application of the CDC Ebola Response Modeling Tool to Disease Predictions, *Epidemics* 22 (March 2018): 22–28.

5.   Carrie F. Nielsen et al., "Improving Burial Practices and Cemetery Management During an Ebola Virus Disease Epidemic—Sierra Leone, 2014," *Morbidity and Mortality Weekly Report* 64, no. 1 (January 16, 2015): 20–27. Safer burial practices were particularly important because corpses have an extraordinarily high viral load and traditional burial practices in the region included washing, dressing, holding, and sometimes kissing the body.

6.   Samantha Power, *The Education of an Idealist: A Memoir* (New York: Dey Street Books, 2019), 406.

7.   Thomas R. Frieden and Inger K. Damon, "Ebola in West Africa—CDC's Role in Epidemic Detection, Control, and Prevention," *Emerging Infectious Diseases* 21, no. 11 (November 1, 2015): 1897–1905.

8.   John Graunt, *Natural and Political Observations Made Upon the Bills of Mortality* (1662; reprinted, Baltimore, MD: The Johns Hopkins Press, 1939). Disease classification has become more precise but perhaps less descriptive in the past 360 years. Graunt's tables included one poor soul who died from fright and eleven who died from grief.

9.   Winslow, *The Life of Hermann M. Biggs.*

10. Amy L. Fairchild et al., "Ethics of Public Health Surveillance: New Guidelines," *Lancet Public Health* 2, no. 8 (August 1, 2017): e348–349; Amy Fairchild, Ronald Bayer, and James Colgrove, "Privacy and Public Health Surveillance: The Enduring Tension," *AMA Journal of Ethics* 9, no. 12 (December 1, 2007): 838–841.

11. Julie Myers et al., "Privacy and Public Health at Risk: Public Health Confidentiality in the Digital Age," *American Journal of Public Health* 98, no. 5 (May 1, 2008): 793–801; Office for Civil Rights, *Breach Portal: Notice to the Secretary of HHS Breach of Unsecured Protected Health Information* (August 8, 2024), distributed by the U.S. Department of Health and Human Services, https://ocrportal.hhs.gov/ocr/breach/breach_report.jsf. Reported breaches of health care data have been much more common than of public health data, perhaps because of the larger volume of data collected by health care facilities and perhaps because public health has had a long-standing practice of protecting confidentiality.

12. Michelle A. Jorden et al., "Evidence for Limited Early Spread of COVID-19 Within the United States, January–February 2020," *Morbidity and Mortality Weekly Report* 69, no. 22 (June 5, 2020): 680–684.

13. Many forms of surveillance track diseases and health trends. Surveillance can be active, in which staff proactively seek the information, or passive, relying on reports from doctors, laboratories, and health care facilities. Sentinel surveillance tracks specific communities or facilities and, although not representative, is an efficient way to track trends over time. Monitoring symptoms rather than diseases, known as syndromic surveillance and discussed in chapter 6, can find an outbreak even when we don't know the cause. Surveys—by phone, in person, or through examination—are essential to understand broader trends. Recent advances let us understand drug-resistance and molecular patterns. Newer methods, including analysis of internet searches, online respondent panels, social media posts, and use of artificial intelligence, may make it possible to spot health trends more promptly.

14. William Farr, *Vital Statistics: A Memorial Volume of Selections from the Reports and Writings of William Far, 1807–1883* (Metuchen, NJ: Offices of the Sanitary Institute, 1975), 123.

15. Kathryn Foti et al., "Hypertension Awareness, Treatment, and Control in US Adults: Trends in the Hypertension Control Cascade by Population Subgroup (National Health and Nutrition Examination Survey, 1999–2016)," *American Journal of Epidemiology* 188, no. 12 (October 15, 2019): 2165–2174.

16. Bruce Lanphear, Ana Navas-Acien, and David C Bellinger, "Lead Poisoning," *New England Journal of Medicine* 391, no. 17 (October 30, 2024): 1621–1631; Rick Nevin, "How Lead Exposure Relates to Temporal Changes in IQ, Violent Crime, and Unwed Pregnancy," *Environmental Research* 83, no. 1 (May 1, 2000): 1–22; John Paul Wright et al., "Association of Prenatal and Childhood Blood Lead Concentrations with Criminal Arrests in Early Adulthood," *PLOS Medicine* 5, no. 5 (May 27, 2008): e101.

17. Vitruvius, *The Ten Books on Architecture*, trans. Morris Hicky Morgan (Cambridge, MA: Harvard University Press, 1914), book VIII.

18. Jerome O. Nriagu, "Saturnine Gout among Roman Aristocrats," *New England Journal of Medicine* 308, no. 11 (March 17, 1983): 660–663.

19. Médecins Sans Frontières (MSF) International, "Nigeria: Prevention Is Key to Stop Children from Dying of Lead Poisoning," February 7, 2022, https://www.msf.org/nigeria-prevention -key-stop-children-dying-lead-poisoning; Carrie A. Dooyema et al., "Outbreak of Fatal Childhood Lead Poisoning Related to Artisanal Gold Mining in Northwestern Nigeria, 2010," *Environmental Health Perspectives* 120, no. 4 (December 20, 2011): 601–607.

20. Upton Sinclair, *The Jungle* (New York: Doubleday, Page & Co., 1906). In the 1890s, Sinclair confidently predicted to Hamilton that the next president would be a socialist; Eugene Debs, socialist candidate for president, received 6 percent of the vote in 1912.

21. Alice Hamilton, *Exploring the Dangerous Trades: The Autobiography of Alice Hamilton, MD* (Boston: Little, Brown, and Co., 1943), 80.

22. Hamilton, *Dangerous Trades*, 3.

23. Hamilton, *Dangerous Trades*, 12.

24. Barbara Sicherman, *Alice Hamilton: A Life in Letters* (Cambridge, MA: Harvard University Press, 1984), 160–161. The foreman of a factory with egregious exposures to lead dismissed the possibility that his factory was causing any health problem, and, if it was, blamed it on ignorant foreign workers. Her letter is a model of tact and diplomacy. Her lifelong, ardent support for immigrants and immigrant rights—which earned her years of FBI surveillance— give context to her comments below, which are meant to preempt the foreman's objections to her recommendations. To quote from her May 22, 1922, letter:

> "My Dear Mr. Foster,
>
> I have just been writing to [the secretary and treasurer of the company] about our conversation of last Friday, as he asked me to put my recommendations down on paper. Now I want to write to you also, because I feel that you are really the one upon whom the reforms depend. The factory which is safe and clean, is the factory which has a foreman who wishes it to be safe and clean. He is the most important factor, for he is there all the time. . . .
>
> As long as your roller room has piles of white lead on the floor and in open trucks, you will always be having lead poisoning. You see you will never be able to make your men careful under those circumstances. . . . I know two white lead factories, old ones at that, where you would not know what was being made in the place, where the floor is so clean you could eat your dinner off it. . . .
>
> I have been able to find only three cases [of lead poisoning at a nearby factory with better practices] for 1910, and twenty-seven from [your factory], yet both factories employ about the same number of men. . . .
>
> It is slow work and difficult to train a lot of foreigners to take care of themselves, but I know you can do it and I am sure there is no man in the white lead business who is more genuinely anxious to protect his men than you are."

25. David Rosner and Gerald Markowitz, "A 'Gift of God'? The Public Health Controversy over Leaded Gasoline during the 1920s," *American Journal of Public Health* 75, no. 4 (April 1, 1985): 344–352.

26. Alice Hamilton, "What Price Safety: Tetra-Ethyl Lead Reveals a Flaw in Our Defenses," *Journal of Occupational Medicine* 14, no. 2 (1972): 98–100, previously published in *Survey Midmonthly* 54, no. 6 (June 15, 1925). Through the 1950s, Dr. Hamilton believed that a study done following the brief pause in production of leaded gasoline had exonerated it and cited use of leaded gasoline as a positive example of a pause followed by appropriate use. It was only later that the extent of harm became clear and that the study cited by Dr. Hamilton and used by industry was deeply flawed.

27. Rosner and Markowitz, "A 'Gift of God'?," 349.

28. Rosner and Markowitz, "A 'Gift of God'?," 349.

29. Kathryn B. Egan et al., "Blood Lead Levels in U.S. Children Ages 1–11 Years, 1976–2016," *Environmental Health Perspectives* 129, no. 3 (March 1, 2021): 37003; U.S. Centers for Disease Control and Prevention (CDC), "National Childhood Blood Lead Surveillance Data," accessed March 8, 2025, https://www.cdc.gov/lead-prevention/php/data/national-surveillance-data.html.

30. Herbert L. Needleman et al., "Deficits in Psychologic and Classroom Performance of Children with Elevated Dentine Lead Levels," *New England Journal of Medicine* 300, no. 13 (March 29, 1979): 689–695. Lead paint contributed to the elevated lead levels, although lead in gasoline caused more widespread contamination.

31. International Labour Office, *White Lead: Data Collected by the International Labour Office in Regard to the Use of White Lead in the Painting Industry*, Studies and Reports Series F, no. 11 (Geneva: International Labour Office, 1927), https://www.ilo.org/public/libdoc/ilo/ILO-SR/ILO-SR_F11_engl.pdf.

32. E. R. Hayhurst and N. C. Dysart, "Industrial Hygiene and Occupational Diseases," *American Journal of Public Health* 13, no. 4 (April 1, 1923): 337–341; "Ratifications of CO13—White Lead (Painting) Convention, 1921 (No. 13)," International Labour Organization, *Ratifications by Conventions* (August 31, 1923), https://www.ilo.org/dyn/normlex/en/f?p=1000:11300:0::NO:11300:P11300_INSTRUMENT_ID:312158.

33. Rosner and Markowitz, "A 'Gift of God'?," 344.

34. Timothy Dignam et al., "Control of Lead Sources in the United States, 1970–2017: Public Health Progress and Current Challenges to Eliminating Lead Exposure," *Journal of Public Health Management and Practice* 25, no. 1 (January 1, 2019): S13–22.

35. CDC, "National Childhood Blood Lead Surveillance Data."

36. Katarzyna Kordas et al., "Lead Exposure in Low and Middle-Income Countries: Perspectives and Lessons on Patterns, Injustices, Economics, and Politics," *International Journal of Environmental Research and Public Health* 15, no. 11 (October 24, 2018): 2351.

37. Benjamin Bowe et al., "Burden of Cause-Specific Mortality Associated With PM2.5 Air Pollution in the United States," *JAMA Network Open* 2, no. 11 (November 20, 2019): e1915834.

38. Richard P. Feynman, "There's Plenty of Room at the Bottom," *Engineering and Science* 23, no. 5 (1960): 22–36, accessed March 8, 2025, https://resolver.caltech.edu/Caltech ES:23.5.1960Bottom.

39. Cristina Buzea, Ivan Pacheco, and Kevin Robbie, "Nanomaterials and Nanoparticles: Sources and Toxicity," *Biointerphases* 2, no. 4 (December 1, 2007): MR17–71; *Approaches to Safe Nanotechnology: Managing the Health and Safety Concerns Associated with Engineered Nanomaterials* (Department of Health and Human Services, Centers for Disease Control and Prevention, National Institute for Occupational Safety and Health, 2009); Lihui Xuan et al., "Nanoparticles-Induced Potential Toxicity on Human Health: Applications, Toxicity Mechanisms, and Evaluation Models," *MedComm* 4, no. 4 (July 14, 2023): e327.

40. Raffaele Marfella et al., "Microplastics and Nanoplastics in Atheromas and Cardiovascular Events," *New England Journal of Medicine* 390, no. 10 (March 7, 2024): 900–910.

41. Linda G. Kahn et al., "Endocrine-Disrupting Chemicals: Implications for Human Health," *Lancet Diabetes & Endocrinology* 8, no. 8 (July 21, 2020): 703–718.

42. Tracey J. Woodruff, "Health Effects of Fossil Fuel–Derived Endocrine Disruptors," *New England Journal of Medicine* 390, no. 10 (March 7, 2024): 922–933.

43. Sharon Lerner, "How 3M Discovered, Then Concealed, the Dangers of Forever Chemicals," *The New Yorker*, May 20, 2024, https://www.newyorker.com/magazine/2024/05/27/3m-forever-chemicals-pfas-pfos-toxic.

44. National Center for Environmental Health, *National Report on Human Exposure to Environmental Chemicals* (Atlanta, GA: U.S. Department of Health and Human Services, U.S. Centers for Disease Control and Prevention, National Center for Environmental Health, March 2024), accessed March 8, 2025, https://www.cdc.gov/environmental-exposure-report/about/index.html.

45. Hamilton, "What Price Safety," 99.

46. Farzad Mostashari et al., "Smoking Practices in New York City: The Use of a Population-Based Survey to Guide Policy-Making and Programming," *Journal of Urban Health* 82, no. 1 (February 28, 2005): 58–70. We were able to estimate trends of the prior decade by obtaining New York City–specific data from a state-wide survey. There were few respondents in New York City; by combining data in three-year brackets we could estimate tobacco use rates.

47. Thomas R. Frieden et al., "Adult Tobacco Use Levels after Intensive Tobacco Control Measures: New York City, 2002–2003," *American Journal of Public Health* 95, no. 6 (June 1, 2005): 1016–1023.

48. J. A. Ellis et al., "Decline in Smoking Prevalence—New York City, 2002–2006," *Morbidity and Mortality Weekly Report* 56, no. 24 (June 22, 2007): 604–608.

49. Terry Pechacek et al., *Best Practices for Comprehensive Tobacco Control Programs—August 1999* (Atlanta, GA: U.S. Department of Health and Human Services, U.S. Centers for Disease

Control and Prevention, National Center for Chronic Disease Prevention and Health Promotion, Office on Smoking and Health, August 1999).

50. Ellis et al., "Decline in Smoking Prevalence."

51. Edward Tufte, *Seeing with Fresh Eyes: Meaning, Space, Data, Truth* (Cheshire, CT: Graphics Press, 2020), 81.

52. Ahmed Jamal et al., "Tobacco Product Use Among Middle and High School Students—National Youth Tobacco Survey, United States, 2024," *Morbidity and Mortality Weekly Report* 73, no. 41 (October 17, 2024): 917–924.

CHAPTER 2

1. Neil K. Mehta, Leah Abrams, and Mikko Myrskylä, "US Life Expectancy Stalls Due to Cardiovascular Disease, Not Drug Deaths," *Proceedings of the National Academy of Sciences of the United States of America* 117, no. 13 (March 16, 2020): 6998–7000.

2. George A. Mensah et al., "Decline in Cardiovascular Mortality," *Circulation Research* 120, no. 2 (January 20, 2017): 366–380.

3. Alex Hollingsworth and Ivan Rudik, "The Effect of Leaded Gasoline on Elderly Mortality: Evidence from Regulatory Exemptions," *American Economic Journal: Economic Policy* 13, no. 3 (July 27, 2021): 345–373.

4. Million Hearts, "Costs & Consequences," U.S. Centers for Disease Control and Prevention, February 26, 2021, accessed March 8, 2025, https://millionhearts.hhs.gov/learn-prevent /cost-consequences.html.

5. Thomas R. Frieden and Donald M. Berwick, "The 'Million Hearts' Initiative—Preventing Heart Attacks and Strokes," *New England Journal of Medicine* 365 (September 29, 2011): e27.

6. Matthew Ritchey et al., *Million Hearts: 2012–2016 Final Report Addendum* (Washington, DC: U.S. Department of Health and Human Services, 2020), https://millionhearts.hhs.gov /files/MH_final_report_addendum_2020.pdf.

7. Geoffrey Rose, *The Strategy of Preventive Medicine* (Oxford: Oxford University Press, 1992), 47, 109.

8. Rose, *Preventive Medicine*, 59.

9. Thomas A. Farley et al., "Deaths Preventable in the U.S. by Improvements in Use of Clinical Preventive Services," *American Journal of Preventive Medicine* 30, no. 6 (June 2010): 600–609.

10. Paul Muntner et al., "Trends in Blood Pressure Control among US Adults with Hypertension, 1999–2000 to 2017–2018," *JAMA* 324, no. 12 (September 22, 2020): 1190.

11. Swati Sakhuja et al., "Reasons for Uncontrolled Blood Pressure among US Adults: Data from the US National Health and Nutrition Examination Survey," *Hypertension* 78, no. 5 (November 1, 2021): 1567–1576.

12. Marc G. Jaffe and Joseph D. Young, "The Kaiser Permanente Northern California Story: Improving Hypertension Control from 44% to 90% in 13 Years (2000 to 2013)," *Journal of Clinical Hypertension* 18, no. 4 (March 3, 2016): 260–261.

13. Rosner and Markowitz, "A 'Gift of God'?," 347.

14. Reinskje Talhout et al., "Cigarette Design Features: Effects on Emission Levels, User Perception, and Behavior," *Tobacco Regulatory Science* 4, no. 1 (November 30, 2017): 592–604; Selvin H. Edwards et al., "Tobacco-Specific Nitrosamines in the Tobacco and Mainstream Smoke of U.S. Commercial Cigarettes," *Chemical Research in Toxicology* 30, no. 2 (November 14, 2016): 540–551.

15. Richard D. Hurt and Channing R. Robertson, "Prying Open the Door to the Tobacco Industry's Secrets About Nicotine," *JAMA* 280, no. 13 (October 7, 1998): 1173.

16. C. J. Shepperd, "The Sensory Enhancement of the Initial Puffs of Low Tar Products Using an Alkaline Additive," December 16, 1993, Product Design MSA Collection, UCSF Industry Documents Library, https://www.industrydocuments.ucsf.edu/docs/hgxk0037; Christina Vaughan Watson et al., "Method for the Determination of Ammonium in Cigarette Tobacco Using Ion Chromatography," *Regulatory Toxicology and Pharmacology* 72, no. 2 (May 2, 2015): 266–270.

17. Reinskje Talhout, Antoon Opperhuizen, and Jan G.C. Van Amsterdam, "Sugars as Tobacco Ingredient: Effects on Mainstream Smoke Composition," *Food and Chemical Toxicology* 44, no. 11 (July 9, 2006): 1789–1798.

18. Robert J. Wickham, "The Biological Impact of Menthol on Tobacco Dependence," *Nicotine & Tobacco Research* 22, no. 10 (December 18, 2019): 1676–1684; U.S. Food and Drug Administration (FDA), Department of Health and Human Services, "21 CFR Part 1162: Proposed Rule," *Federal Register* 87, no. 26454 (May 5, 2022): 26454–26456, Docket No. FDA-2021-N-1349, RIN 0910-AI60, https://www.federalregister.gov/documents/2022/05/04/2022-08994/tobacco-product-standard-for-menthol-in-cigarettes.

19. Thomas R. Frieden and Drew E. Blakeman, "The Dirty Dozen: 12 Myths That Undermine Tobacco Control," *American Journal of Public Health* 95, no. 9 (September 1, 2005): 1500–1505.

20. Ahmad El-Hellani, Theodore L. Wagener, and Marielle C. Brinkman, "Reengineering Addiction—the Tobacco Industry's Potential Response to a Nicotine Standard for Cigarettes," *New England Journal of Medicine*, May 4, 2024; Hurt and Robertson, "Prying Open the Door"; Wallace B. Pickworth et al., "Nicotine Absorption from Smokeless Tobacco Modified to Adjust pH," *Journal of Addiction Research & Therapy* 5, no. 3 (January 1, 2014); FDA, "21 CFR Part 1162."

21. U.S. Congress, House Committee on Energy and Commerce, Subcommittee on Health and the Environment, "Regulation of Tobacco Products (Part 1)," 103rd Congress, 2nd session, April 14, 1994.

22. *The Health Consequences of Smoking—50 Years of Progress: A Report of the Surgeon General* (Atlanta, GA: U.S. Department of Health and Human Services, 2014); World Health Organization (WHO), "Tobacco: Key Facts," July 31, 2023, https://www.who.int/news-room/fact-sheets/detail/tobacco.

23. Margaret Ramirez, "Anti-Smoking Push Faces Budget Crunch," *Newsday*, February 15, 2002.

24. U.S. Centers for Disease Control and Prevention, "Tobacco Industry Spending," September 3, 2024, accessed March 8, 2025, https://www.cdc.gov/tobacco/php/tobacco-industry-spending/index.html.

25. Richard W. Pollay, "Promises, Promises: Self-Regulation of US Cigarette Broadcast Advertising in the 1960s," *Tobacco Control* 3, no. 2 (1994): 134–144.

26. Rose, *Preventive Medicine*, 90, 135, 161.

27. Frankie Edozien, "A Pain in the Ash; Bloomberg Signs Smoke Ban into Law," *New York Post*, December 31, 2002, https://nypost.com/2002/12/31/a-pain-in-the-ash-bloomberg-signs-smoke-ban-into-law/.

28. Christina Chang et al., "The New York City Smoke-Free Air Act: Second-Hand Smoke as a Worker Health and Safety Issue," *American Journal of Industrial Medicine* 46, no. 2 (July 19, 2004): 188–195.

29. Dana A. Shea and Sarah A. Lister, *The BioWatch Program: Detection of Bioterrorism* (Congressional Research Service, 2003), https://crsreports.congress.gov/product/details?prodcode=RL32152.

30. Shea and Lister, *BioWatch Program*.

31. U.S. Government Accountability Office (GAO), "Information Technology: Federal Agencies Face Challenges in Implementing Initiatives to Improve Public Health Infrastructure," June 10, 2005, https://www.gao.gov/products/gao-05-308; GAO, "Biosurveillance: DHS Should Reevaluate Mission Need and Alternatives before Proceeding with BioWatch Generation-3 Acquisition," September 10, 2012, https://www.gao.gov/products/gao-12-810; GAO, "Biosurveillance: Observations on the Cancellation of BioWatch Gen-3 and Future Considerations for the Program," June 10, 2014, https://www.gao.gov/products/gao-14-267t; GAO, "Biosurveillance: DHS Should Not Pursue BioWatch Upgrades or Enhancements until System Capabilities Are Established," October 23, 2015, https://www.gao.gov/products/gao-16-99; GAO, "Biodefense: DHS Exploring New Methods to Replace BioWatch and Could Benefit from Additional Guidance," May 20, 2021, https://www.gao.gov/products/gao-21-292; GAO, "Biodefense: Actions Needed to Address Long-Standing Challenges," March 9, 2023, https://www.gao.gov/products/gao-23-106476.

32. George Ainslie and Nick Haslam, "Hyperbolic Discounting," in *Choice Over Time, ed. George Loewenstein and Jon Elster* (New York: Russell Sage Foundation, 1992), 57–92.

33. John Cawley and Christopher J. Ruhm, "The Economics of Risky Health Behaviors," in *Handbook of Health Economics*, ed. Mark V. Pauly, Thomas G. McGuire, and Pedro P. Barros (Elsevier, 2011), 95–199; Paul Slovic, "Understanding Perceived Risk: 1978–2015,"

Environment Science and Policy for Sustainable Development 58, no. 1 (December 31, 2015): 25–29.

34. Haim Omer and Nahman Alon, "The Continuity Principle: A Unified Approach to Disaster and Trauma," *American Journal of Community Psychology* 22, no. 2 (April 1, 1994): 273–287.

35. National Conference on High Blood Pressure Education, *Report of Proceedings* (Bethesda, MD: National Institutes of Health, 1973), conference address by Jeremiah Stamler, MD, "High Blood Pressure in the U.S.—An Overview of the Problem and Challenge," January 15, 1973; J. T. Hart, "Rule of Halves: Implications of Increasing Diagnosis and Reducing Dropout for Future Workload and Prescribing Costs in Primary Care," *British Journal of General Practice* 42, no. 356 (March 1, 1992): 116–119.

36. Rachel O. Reid, Cheryl L. Damberg, and Mark W. Friedberg, "Primary Care Spending in the Fee-for-Service Medicare Population," *JAMA Internal Medicine* 179, no. 7 (July 1, 2019): 977.

37. Kari Redfield, "Physician Salary Report 2023: Physician Income Continues to Rise," *Weatherby* (blog), August 30, 2023, https://weatherbyhealthcare.com/blog/annual-physician-salary-report-2023.

38. Ainslie and Haslam, "Hyperbolic Discounting," 57–92.

39. Aaron T. Beck, *Cognitive Therapy and the Emotional Disorders* (Madison, CT: International Universities Press, 1972).

CHAPTER 3

1. Michael D. Shear and Mark Landler, "Amid Assurances on Ebola, Obama Is Said to Seethe," *New York Times*, October 18, 2014, https://www.nytimes.com/2014/10/18/us/amid-assurances-on-ebola-obama-is-said-to-seethe.html.

2. Mary J. Choi et al., "A Case of Lassa Fever Diagnosed at a Community Hospital—Minnesota 2014," *Open Forum Infectious Diseases* 5, no. 7 (July 1, 2018): ofy131.

3. N. Fujita et al., "Imported Case of Marburg Hemorrhagic Fever—Colorado, 2008," *Morbidity and Mortality Weekly Report* 303, no. 5 (2010): 413–415.

4. The HIV epidemic changed this dynamic. Rather than one in ten, at least half of immunosuppressed people infected with the tuberculosis bacteria develop active disease. This susceptibility results in explosive spread of tuberculosis in communities with a high prevalence of HIV, as occurred in New York City hospitals and in countries around the world, particularly in Africa.

5. Bibha Dhungel et al., "Reliability of Early Estimates of the Basic Reproduction Number of COVID-19: A Systematic Review and Meta-Analysis," *International Journal of Environmental Research and Public Health* 19, no. 18 (September 15, 2022): 11613.

6. Using a reproductive number to track infectious diseases is easy to understand—how many people each case infects—but has limitations. It's hard to calculate, is based on untestable

assumptions, and is just a rough estimate. It changes over time and can be calculated in different ways. Despite these limitations, the concept can be useful if a single model is used over time. That way, the trend can indicate, with some delay, whether things are going in the right direction—whether disease spread is accelerating or decelerating, indicating whether control measures are working.

There's a better way to assess and improve control. Transmission risk results from three independent factors: how long people are infectious, how many people they come into contact with, and how likely infection spreads during those contacts. It's more useful to measure and reduce each of these risks through faster diagnosis, effective isolation, and reducing spread during exposures. To reduce the infectious period, decrease the delay between patients feeling sick and getting isolated. To reduce the number of contacts, determine the contact index—the average number of contacts each patient has—and reduce it by faster and better isolation of infectious patients. And to reduce the likelihood of spread during contact, measure infection among exposed people and reduce it by decreasing risky activities.

7. Paul L. Delamater et al., "Complexity of the Basic Reproduction Number (R_0)," *Emerging Infectious Diseases* 25, no. 1 (January 1, 2019): 1–4.

8. Riley et al., "Aerial Dissemination of Pulmonary Tuberculosis."

9. It's more accurate to speak of superspreading events than superspreading people (Thomas R. Frieden and Christopher T. Lee, "Identifying and Interrupting Superspreading Events—Implications for Control of Severe Acute Respiratory Syndrome Coronavirus 2," *Emerging Infectious Diseases* 26, no. 6 [June 1, 2020]: 1059–1066). New York City found and stopped a tuberculosis outbreak that began in a high school choir—singing is an efficient way to spread a respiratory infection. One student who sang in the choir while ill caused at least six secondary cases and many more infections, including among students who used the classroom the period *after* choir, indicating that infectious tuberculosis droplets remained airborne for hours (Rita Washko et al., "Tuberculosis Transmission in a High School Choir," *Journal of School Health* 68, no. 6 [August 1, 1998]: 256–259). Similarly, on March 10, 2020, sixty-one members of a choir in Skagit County, Washington State, gathered for rehearsal. One was ill with COVID. Three weeks after the rehearsal, fifty-three of the sixty-one choir members had COVID, three required hospitalization, and two died (Lea Hamner et al., "High SARS-CoV-2 Attack Rate Following Exposure at a Choir Practice—Skagit County, Washington, March 2020," *Morbidity and Mortality Weekly Report* 69, no. 19 [May 15, 2020]: 606–610).

10. Preventing superspreading is easier said than done. Many superspreading events occur in health care facilities. Superspreading highlights the need for fast, expert public health work to prevent spread by finding cases and infected contacts quickly. More importantly, by recognizing where a disease is spreading, communities can prevent future superspreading events. Safer hospitals, canceled choir practice, and, when appropriate, closed bars and nightclubs are all effective, rigorous, data-driven approaches to protect people from explosive and potentially deadly lung infections. Chapter 8 reviews the ethics and practicality of such measures.

11. Edwin A. Mitchell et al., "Results from the 1st Year of the New Zealand Cot Death Study," *New Zealand Medical Journal* 104, no. 906 (1992): 71–76.

12. Edwin A. Mitchell in conversation with the author, April 24, 2024.

13. Mitchell et al., "Results from the 1st Year of the New Zealand Cot Death Study."

14. Edwin A. Mitchell, Lynn Hutchison, and Alistair W Stewart, "The Continuing Decline in SIDS Mortality," *Archives of Disease in Childhood* 92 (2007): 625–626.

15. Angus Deaton and Nancy Cartwright, "Understanding and Misunderstanding Randomized Controlled Trials," *Social Science & Medicine* 210 (August 1, 2018): 2–21.

16. Jessie R. Chung et al., "Seasonal Effectiveness of Live Attenuated and Inactivated Influenza Vaccine," *Pediatrics* 137, no. 2 (February 1, 2016): e20153279.

17. Thomas R. Frieden, "Evidence for Health Decision Making—Beyond Randomized, Controlled Trials," *New England Journal of Medicine* 377, no. 5 (August 3, 2017): 465–475.

18. George W. Comstock, Verna T. Livesay, and Shirley F. Woolpert, "The Prognosis of a Positive Tuberculin Reaction in Childhood and Adolescence," *American Journal of Epidemiology* 99, no. 2 (February 1, 1974): 131–138.

19. George W. Comstock, "Tuberculosis: Is the Past Once Again Prologue?," *American Journal of Public Health* 84, no. 11 (November 1, 1994): 1729–1731.

20. Michael Schulson, "Are Evidence-Based Medicine and Public Health Incompatible?," *Undark*, February 21, 2024, https://undark.org/2024/02/21/evidence-based-medicine/.

21. An example of an erroneous review is Tom Jefferson et al., "Physical Interventions to Interrupt or Reduce the Spread of Respiratory Viruses," *Cochrane Library* 2023, no. 4 (January 30, 2023): CD006207. For critique, see Shama Cash-Goldwasser et al., "Masks During Pandemics Caused by Respiratory Pathogens—Evidence and Implications for Action," *JAMA Network Open* 6, no. 10 (October 31, 2023): e2339443.

22. Naveed Sattar and David Preiss, "Reverse Causality in Cardiovascular Epidemiological Research," *Circulation* 135, no. 24 (June 13, 2017): 2369–2372.

23. Laura K. Cobb, Thomas R. Frieden, and Lawrence J. Appel, "No U-turn on Sodium Reduction," *Journal of Clinical Hypertension* 22, no. 11 (August 29, 2020): 2156–2160.

24. Bente Deutch et al., "Traditional and Modern Greenlandic Food—Dietary Composition, Nutrients and Contaminants," *Science of the Total Environment* 384, no. 1–3 (October 1, 2007): 106–119.

25. Hyuna Sung et al., "Global Cancer Statistics 2020: GLOBOCAN Estimates of Incidence and Mortality Worldwide for 36 Cancers in 185 Countries," *CA: A Cancer Journal for Clinicians* 71, no. 3 (February 4, 2021): 209–249.

26. Laszlo Tabar et al., "Mammography Service Screening and Mortality in Breast Cancer Patients: 20-Year Follow-Up Before and After Introduction of Screening," *The Lancet* 361, no. 9367 (April 1, 2003): 1405–1410.

27. Søren Riis Christiansen, Philippe Autier, and Henrik Støvring, "Change in Effectiveness of Mammography Screening with Decreasing Breast Cancer Mortality: A Population-based Study," *European Journal of Public Health* 32, no. 4 (June 23, 2022): 630–635.

28. Farley et al., "Deaths Preventable in the U.S."

29. Davidson R. Gwatkin and Alex Ergo, "Universal Health Coverage: Friend or Foe of Health Equity?" *Lancet* 377, no. 9784 (June 25, 2011): 2160–2161.

30. Hans Rosling, *Factfulness: Ten Reasons We're Wrong About the World—and Why Things Are Better Than You Think* (New York: Flatiron Books, 2018), 181.

31. Thomas R. Frieden, "A Framework for Public Health Action: The Health Impact Pyramid," *American Journal of Public Health* 100, no. 4 (April 1, 2010): 590–595.

32. Thomas R. Frieden, "Tuberculosis Control and Social Change," *American Journal of Public Health* 84, no. 11 (November 1, 1994): 1721–1723.

33. Andrew J. Shattock et al., "Contribution of Vaccination to Improved Survival and Health: Modelling 50 Years of the Expanded Programme on Immunization," *Lancet* 403, no. 10441 (May 1, 2024): 2307–2316.

34. The relationship between socioeconomic status and hypertension isn't straightforward. In the United States, Europe, and China, people with lower income or less education have higher rates of hypertension. In parts of Africa and Asia, higher income was traditionally associated with higher body weight and, in some communities, higher rates of hypertension. In these regions, lower income and lower education level increasingly correlate with hypertension in most communities. See Bing Leng et al., "Socioeconomic Status and Hypertension," *Journal of Hypertension* 33, no. 2 (December 5, 2014): 221–229; Tao Luo et al., "Relationship Between Socioeconomic Status and Hypertension Incidence Among Adults in Southwest China: A Population-based Cohort Study," *BMC Public Health* 24, no. 1 (May 2, 2024): 1211; Aishat Mustapha et al., "Hypertension and Socioeconomic Status in South Central Uganda: A Population-Based Cohort Study," *Global Heart* 17, no. 1 (January 1, 2022): 3; Gulam Muhammed Al Kibria et al., "Clustering of Hypertension, Diabetes and Overweight/ Obesity According to Socioeconomic Status Among Bangladeshi Adults," *Journal of Biosocial Science* 53, no. 2 (March 9, 2020): 157–166; City of New York, *NYC Health and Nutrition Examination Survey*, accessed March 8, 2025, https://www.nyc.gov/site/doh/data/data-sets /new-york-city-health-and-nutrition-examination-survey-documentation.page.

35. Bruce Neal et al., "Effect of Salt Substitution on Cardiovascular Events and Death," *New England Journal of Medicine* 385, no. 12 (September 16, 2021): 1067–1077; "FDA Issues Voluntary Sodium Reduction Targets for Food Industry," Center for Science in the Public Interest, April 5, 2023, https://www.cspinet.org/statement/fda-issues-voluntary-sodium -reduction-targets-food-industry; Michael F. Jacobson, *Salt Wars: The Battle Over the Biggest Killer in the American Diet* (Cambridge, MA: MIT Press, 2020).

36. Nicole Ide et al., "Priority Actions to Advance Population Sodium Reduction," *Nutrients* 12, no. 9 (August 22, 2020): 2543; Lindsey Smith Taillie et al., "Decreases in Purchases of

Energy, Sodium, Sugar, and Saturated Fat 3 Years After Implementation of the Chilean Food Labeling and Marketing Law: An Interrupted Time Series Analysis," *PLOS Medicine* 21, no. 9 (September 27, 2024): e1004463.

37. Johanna M. Geleijnse et al., "Long-Term Effects of Neonatal Sodium Restriction on Blood Pressure," *Hypertension* 29, no. 4 (April 1, 1997): 913–917. Erratum in *Hypertension* 29, no. 5 (May 1997): 1211.

38. Davor Vukadinović et al., "Effects of Catheter-Based Renal Denervation in Hypertension: A Systematic Review and Meta-Analysis," *Circulation*, October 2, 2024; Akshay S. Desai et al., "Zilebesiran, an RNA Interference Therapeutic Agent for Hypertension," *New England Journal of Medicine* 389, no. 3 (July 19, 2023): 228–238.

39. Sara Pedron et al., "The Effect of Population-Based Blood Pressure Screening on Long-Term Cardiometabolic Morbidity and Mortality in Germany: A Regression Discontinuity Analysis," *PLOS Medicine* 19, no. 12 (December 27, 2022): e1004151; Hyuncheol Bryant Kim, Suejin A. Lee, and Wilfredo Lim, "Knowing Is Not Half the Battle: Impacts of Information from the National Health Screening Program in Korea," *Journal of Health Economics* 65 (March 1, 2019): 1–14.

40. Lirije Hyseni et al., "Systematic Review of Dietary Salt Reduction Policies: Evidence for an Effectiveness Hierarchy?," *PLOS One* 12, no. 5 (May 18, 2017): e0177535 and Alma J. Adler et al., "Reduced Dietary Salt for the Prevention of Cardiovascular Disease," *Cochrane Library* 2017, no. 7 (December 18, 2014).

41. Ben Lacey et al., "Age-Specific Association Between Blood Pressure and Vascular and Non-Vascular Chronic Diseases in 0·5 Million Adults in China: A Prospective Cohort Study," *Lancet Global Health* 6, no. 6 (June 1, 2018): e641–649.

42. The SPRINT Research Group, "A Randomized Trial of Intensive Versus Standard Blood-Pressure Control," *New England Journal of Medicine* 373, no. 22 (November 26, 2015): 2103–2116.

43. Reprinted as: Rudolf Virchow, "Report on the Typhus Epidemic in Upper Silesia," *American Journal of Public Health* 96, no. 12 (December 1, 2006): 2102–2105. See also Rex Taylor and Annelie Rieger, "Medicine as Social Science: Rudolf Virchow on the Typhus Epidemic in Upper Silesia," *International Journal of Health Services* 15, no. 4 (October 1, 1985): 547–559.

44. Thomas R. Frieden, "Six Components Necessary for Effective Public Health Program Implementation," *American Journal of Public Health* 104, no. 1 (January 1, 2014): 17–22.

45. Ian Smith, "What Is DOTS?," in *Toman's Tuberculosis*, ed. by Thomas R. Frieden (Geneva, Switzerland: World Health Organization, 2004), 241. DOTS stood for Directly Observed Treatment, Short-course.

46. WHO, *Global Tuberculosis Report 2023* (Geneva, Switzerland, 2023), https://www.who .int/publications/i/item/9789240083851; Philippe Glaziou, Katherine Floyd, and Mario Raviglione, "Global Epidemiology of Tuberculosis," *Seminars in Respiratory and Critical Care Medicine* 39, no. 3 (June 1, 2018): 271–285. Tuberculosis remains the world's leading cause

of death from an infectious disease. Without an effective vaccine, simpler treatment, and a way to find and treat infection in the people who will develop tuberculosis in the future, progress requires persistence. See: Thomas R. Frieden, Karen F. Brudney, and Anthony D. Harries, "Global Tuberculosis: Perspectives, Prospects, and Priorities," *JAMA* 312, no. 14 (September 5, 2014): 1393–1394.

47. Kelly Henning and Jennifer Ellis, "How Evidence Has Fueled Bloomberg Philanthropies' Work in Tobacco Control," *Health Affairs* (March 26, 2019), https://www.healthaffairs.org /do/10.1377/forefront.20190325.697700/full/.

48. WHO, *Countdown to 2023: WHO 5-Year Milestone Report on Global Trans Fat Elimination 2023* (Geneva, Switzerland, 2024), https://www.who.int/publications/i/item/9789240089549.

49. Hypertension Detection and Follow-up Program Cooperative Group, "Five-Year Findings of the Hypertension Detection and Follow-up Program," *JAMA* 242, no. 23 (December 7, 1979): 2562.

50. John A. Sbarbaro, "Public Health Aspects of Tuberculosis: Supervision of Therapy," *Clinics in Chest Medicine* 1, no. 2 (1980): 253–263.

51. Neo Tapela et al., "Prevalence and Determinants of Hypertension Control Among Almost 100,000 Treated Adults in the UK," *Open Heart* 8, no. 1 (February 1, 2021): e001461; Tim Doran et al., "Pay-for-Performance Programs in Family Practices in the United Kingdom," *New England Journal of Medicine* 355, no. 4 (July 26, 2006): 375–384.

52. Eisuke Nakazawa, Hiroyasu Ino, and Akira Akabayashi, "Chronology of COVID-19 Cases on the Diamond Princess Cruise Ship and Ethical Considerations: A Report from Japan," *Disaster Medicine and Public Health Preparedness* 14, no. 4 (March 24, 2020): 506–513; Lisa Schnirring, "COVID-19 Sickens Over 1,700 Health Workers in China, Killing 6," *CIDRAP*, February 14, 2020, https://www.cidrap.umn.edu/covid-19/covid -19-sickens-over-1700-health-workers-china-killing-6.

53. Kenji Mizumoto et al., "Estimating the Asymptomatic Proportion of Coronavirus Disease 2019 (COVID 19) Cases on Board the Diamond Princess Cruise Ship, Yokohama, Japan, 2020," *Eurosurveillance* 25, no. 10 (March 12, 2020).

54. CDC, "CDC Update on Novel Coronavirus," Transcript for CDC Telebriefing (February 5, 2020), accessed March 8, 2025, https://stacks.cdc.gov/view/cdc/84802.

55. Bill Foege, "Lessons from a Mentor," *Lancet* 382, no. 9899 (October 1, 2013): 1169.

56. CDC, "CDC Update on Novel Coronavirus."

57. "President Trump Talks to Trish Regan Ahead of NH Primary," *Trish Regan Primetime*, FOX News (February 10, 2020).

58. JoAnne Micale Foody, Michael H. Farrell, and Harlan M. Krumholz, "β-Blocker Therapy in Heart Failure," *JAMA* 287, no. 7 (February 20, 2002): 883.

59. Jenny Gold, "Harkin Accuses Administration of 'Robbing Peter to Pay Paul'—KFF Health News," *KFF Health News*, April 11, 2013, https://kffhealthnews.org/news/harkin -accuses-administration-of-robbing-peter-to-pay-paul/.

CHAPTER 4

1. Diego Forni et al., "Analysis of Variola Virus Molecular Evolution Suggests an Old Origin of the Virus Consistent with Historical Records," *Microbial Genomics* 9, no. 1 (January 9, 2023).

2. Elizabeth A. Fenn, "Biological Warfare in Eighteenth-Century North America: Beyond Jeffery Amherst," *Journal of American History* 86, no. 4 (March 1, 2000): 1552–1580.

3. Ann M. Becker, "Smallpox in Washington's Army: Strategic Implications of the Disease during the American Revolutionary War," *The Journal of Military History* 68, no. 2 (January 1, 2004): 381–430.

4. William H. Foege, J. Donald Millar, and John Lane, "Selective Epidemiologic Control in Smallpox Eradication," *American Journal of Epidemiology* 94, no. 4 (October 1, 1971): 311–315. An earlier epidemiologic discovery showed why this strategy works: Vaccinating someone even four to five days after they have been exposed to smallpox will likely protect them. This makes it possible to stop an outbreak even after many people have been exposed—but only if they are found and vaccinated within a few days of exposure.

5. William H. Foege, *House on Fire: The Fight to Eradicate Smallpox* (Berkeley: University of California Press; New York: Milbank Memorial Fund, 2011). One innovation that made smallpox eradication possible is a simple, inexpensive needle with a forked end point (called a bifurcated needle). This allowed the right dose of vaccine to dwell between the tines of the fork. With just a few minutes of training, virtually anyone could learn to use a bifurcated needle and vaccinate safely and successfully.

6. Frank Fenner et al., *Smallpox and Its Eradication* (Geneva, Switzerland: World Health Organization, 1988).

7. John Duffy, *History of Public Health in New York City, 1625–1866*, vol. 1 (New York: Russell Sage Foundation, 1968), xvi.

8. C.-E. A. Winslow, *The Evolution and Significance of the Modern Public Health Campaign* (New Haven, CT: Yale University Press, 1923), 65.

9. Steven Pinker, *The Better Angels of Our Nature: Why Violence Has Declined* (New York: Viking, 2011).

10. Rosling, *Factfulness*, 99.

11. Jonathan Gorstein et al., "Estimating the Health and Economic Benefits of Universal Salt Iodization Programs to Correct Iodine Deficiency Disorders," *Thyroid* 30, no. 12 (December 1, 2020): 1802–1809.

12. Samuel L. Katz and Alan R. Hinman, "Summary and Conclusions: Measles Elimination Meeting, 16–17 March 2000," *Journal of Infectious Diseases* 189 (May 1, 2004): S43–47.

13. Anna A. Minta et al., "Progress toward Measles Elimination—Worldwide, 2000–2022," *Morbidity and Mortality Weekly Report*, 72, no. 46 (November 17, 2023): 1262–1268.

14. Smith, "What Is DOTS?," 241; World Health Organization, *WHO Tuberculosis Programme: Framework for Effective Tuberculosis Control* (Geneva, Switzerland, 1994), https://iris.who .int/handle/10665/58717.

15. World Health Organization, *A Brief History of Tuberculosis Control in India* (Geneva, Switzerland, 2010), https://www.who.int/docs/default-source/documents/tuberculosis /9789241500159-eng.pdf?sfvrsn=48c90fb6_2.

16. G. R. Khatri and Thomas R. Frieden, "The Status and Prospects of Tuberculosis Control in India," *International Journal of Tuberculosis and Lung Disease* 4, no. 3 (March 2000): 193–200.

17. Bent Flyvbjerg and Dan Gardner, *How Big Things Get Done: The Surprising Factors That Determine the Fate of Every Project, from Home Renovations to Space Exploration and Everything in Between* (New York: Currency, 2023).

18. Thomas R. Frieden and G. R. Khatri, "Impact of National Consultants on Successful Expansion of Effective Tuberculosis Control in India," *International Journal of Tuberculosis and Lung Disease* 7, no. 9 (September 2003): 837–841.

19. Rafael Obregón et al., "Achieving Polio Eradication: A Review of Health Communication Evidence and Lessons Learned in India and Pakistan," *Bulletin of the World Health Organization* 87, no. 8 (August 1, 2009): 624–630.

20. Thomas R. Frieden, "Can Tuberculosis Be Controlled?," *Indian Journal of Tuberculosis* 45 (1998): 65–72.

21. Alan Rozanski et al., "Association of Optimism with Cardiovascular Events and All-Cause Mortality," *JAMA Network Open* 2, no. 9 (September 27, 2019): e1912200.

22. Malcolm Gladwell, "The Mosquito Killer," *New Yorker*, July 2, 2001.

23. Tali Sharot, "The Optimism Bias," *Current Biology* 21, no. 23 (December 1, 2011): R941–945.

24. Neil D. Weinstein, "Unrealistic Optimism about Future Life Events," *Journal of Personality and Social Psychology*, 39 no. 5 (1980): 806 820. We also have a negativity bias, which leads us to give more weight to losses; this can undermine the motivation to act.

25. World Health Organization, *Global Report on Hypertension: The Race Against a Silent Killer* (Geneva, Switzerland, 2023), 36–37, https://www.who.int/publications/i/item /9789240081062; Kulpimol Charoendee et al., "Assessment of Population Coverage of Hypertension Screening in Thailand Based on the Effective Coverage Framework," *BMC Health Services Research* 18, no. 1 (March 27, 2018); Thomas R. Frieden et al., "Improved Hypertension Care Requires Measurement and Management in Health Facilities, Not Mass Screening," *Lancet* 405, no. 10490 (May 7, 2025), https://doi.org/10.1016/S0140-6736(25) 00561-6. In contrast, universal measurement of blood pressure among patients attending health facilities—something not routinely done in many lower-income countries—is efficient and effective to diagnose patients and link them to care (see Mogan Kaviprawin and Archana Ramalingam et al., "Missed Opportunities for Detection of Hypertension in Public Health Facilities of 18 Districts in India, 2022," *BMC Public Health* 25 [March 21, 2025]: 1082).

26. Laura Dyrda, "'There Are Billions of Dollars Being Wasted': What CIOs Think of Digital Health Startups," *Becker's Health IT*, July 1, 2022, https://www.beckershospitalreview.com /digital-health/there-are-billions-of-dollars-being-wasted-what-cios-think-of-digital-health -startups.html.

27. Amy Edmonson, *Right Kind of Wrong: The Science of Failing Well* (New York: Atria Books, 2023).

28. Rosling, *Factfulness*, 165.

29. Stephen M. Shortell and Rodney K. McCurdy, "Integrated Health Systems," *Information, Knowledge, Systems Management* 8, no. 1–4 (January 1, 2009): 369–382; Brent C. James and Lucy A. Savitz, "How Intermountain Trimmed Health Care Costs Through Robust Quality Improvement Efforts," *Health Affairs* 30, no. 6 (June 1, 2011): 1185–1191; Leonard Berry and Dan Beckham, "Team-Based Care at Mayo Clinic: A Model for ACOs," *Journal of Healthcare Management* 51, no. 1 (2014): 9–13.

30. Margaret E. Kruk et al., "The Contribution of Primary Care to Health and Health Systems in Low- and Middle-Income Countries: A Critical Review of Major Primary Care Initiatives," *Social Science & Medicine* 70, no. 6 (March 1, 2010): 904–911.

31. David Muhlestein, Tianna Tu, and Carrie H. Colla, "Accountable Care Organizations Are Increasingly Led by Physician Groups Rather Than Hospital Systems," *American Journal of Managed Care* 26, no. 5 (2020): 225–228.

CHAPTER 5

1. Faisal Shuaib et al., "Ebola Virus Disease Outbreak—Nigeria, July–September 2014," *Morbidity and Mortality Weekly Report* 63, no. 39 (2014): 867–872.

2. "Remarks by President Trump, Vice President Pence, and Members of the Coronavirus Task Force in Press Briefing," White House Press Briefing (April 1, 2020), accessed March 8, 2025, https://trumpwhitehouse.archives.gov/briefings-statements/remarks-president-trump-vice -president-pence-members-coronavirus-task-force-press-briefing-5/.

3. Stephen R. Covey, *The 7 Habits of Highly Effective People* (New York: Free Press, 1989).

4. Honing the hypertension treatment algorithm might require quadrant I activities such as convincing a new clinician or policymaker not to change something that's working, quadrant III activities of answering media questions about the regimen, and resisting quadrant IV activities such as detailed analysis of outcomes without an impact on improving the regimen. Quadrant II activities include analyzing the effectiveness of the selected regimen to defend and improve it and implementing research projects to find the most effective, practical, and affordable regimen. The same dynamic is in place for a regular supply of drugs and blood pressure monitors; quadrant II activities might include improving the procurement system, establishing information feedback loops to prevent stock-outs and oversupply, and working with manufacturers to develop products that better meet the needs of health care workers and patients. To promote team-based care, quadrant II activities include documenting superior

outcomes and lower costs of this approach, establishing training and support programs for the allied health staff who implement the program, and supporting organizations of nurses and community health workers to advocate for their roles as part of treatment teams. A particularly important quadrant II activity for patient-friendly services is convincing policymakers that treatment for hypertension should be free of cost to the patient. Any copayments reduce patient adherence and increase the number of strokes and heart attacks that will occur, but eliminating payments requires convincing policymakers to spend more money now to avoid more expenditures and negative health outcomes later. See, for example, Thomas R. Frieden et al., "Unlocking Health Equity by Eliminating Copayments for Essential Antihypertensive Medications," *EClinicalMedicine* 81 (January 30, 2025): 103094. Most current health information systems are cumbersome and ineffective at improving blood pressure control. Another classic quadrant II activity is simplifying indicators and establishing practical electronic systems to empower health care workers to see and improve patient outcomes.

5.   Lucia Brugnara et al., "Strengthening National Public Health Institutes: A Systematic Review on Institution Building in the Public Sector," *Frontiers in Public Health* 11 (May 18, 2023).

6.   James Q. Wilson, *Bureaucracy: What Government Agencies Do and Why They Do It* (New York: Basic Books, 1989), 24.

7.   Wilson, *Bureaucracy*, 375.

8.   Wilson, *Bureaucracy*, 371.

9.   Beth Meyerson, Fred A. Martich, and Gerald P. Naehr, *Ready to Go: The History and Contributions of U.S. Public Health Advisors* (Research Triangle Park, NC: American Social Health Organization, 2008).

10.   Elizabeth W. Etheridge, *Sentinel for Health: A History of the Centers for Disease Control* (Berkeley: University of California Press, 1992), 169.

11.   Atul Gawande, *The Checklist Manifesto: How to Get Things Right* (New York: Metropolitan Books, 2009).

12.   Betty Bard MacDonald, *The Plague and I* (Philadelphia: J.B. Lippincott Co., 1948).

13.   Congressional Budget Office, *Comparing the Compensation of Federal and Private-Sector Employees, 2011 to 2015* (April 25, 2017), https://www.cbo.gov/publication/52637.

14.   International Monetary Fund, *Making Public Investment More Efficient* (Washington, DC: IMF Policy Papers, 2015).

15.   It's possible to further reduce corruption and increase efficiency by improving the purchasing and contracting processes. Purchasing must address not only price but actual functioning and durability. Contracting for services requires finding the right individual or organization, establishing a simple, clear, enforceable contract, and managing the contractor well so their activities are integrated and aligned with the contracting organization, other contractors, and relevant individuals and organizations.

16. Joanne Liu, "MSF President's Remarks to the UN Special Briefing on Ebola," Médecins Sans Frontières (Speech, September 16, 2014), https://www.msf.org/msf-presidents-remarks -un-special-briefing-ebola.

17. Bridget M. Kuehn, "Guinea Worm Disease Eradication Is Within Reach," *JAMA* 326, no. 23 (December 21, 2021): 2353; Norbert W. Brattig, Robert A. Cheke, and Rolf Garms, "Onchocerciasis (River Blindness)—More Than a Century of Research and Control," *Acta Tropica* 218 (June 1, 2021): 105677.

18. Jean-Robert Ioset and Shing Chang, "Drugs for Neglected Diseases Initiative Model of Drug Development for Neglected Diseases: Current Status and Future Challenges," *Future Medicinal Chemistry* 3, no. 11 (September 1, 2011): 1361–1371; Drugs for Neglected Diseases Initiative (DNDi), *DNDi 2022 Annual Report* (October 11, 2023), https://dndi.org /publications/2023/dndi-2022-annual-report/.

CHAPTER 6

1. Brudney and Dobkin, "Resurgent Tuberculosis in New York City."

2. Another approach, still advocated by some groups, is detailed assessment of the patient's risk for bad outcomes before starting treatment. The argument is sophisticated: A patient with a blood pressure of 155/85 who is otherwise healthy has a lower risk of stroke or heart attack than a patient with a blood pressure of 145/80 who smokes, is obese, and has high cholesterol. But in nearly all situations, assessing risk so complicates the diagnosis that many patients who would benefit don't get treated. The disconnect between recommendations and the practical realities of doctors, nurses, pharmacists, and other staff in busy health centers is a major reason for failure of health programs around the world.

   Of course, assessing risk *is* important and can result in better treatment. Some countries and programs establish a lower blood pressure target, such as 130/80, for patients who have both diabetes and hypertension. Risk analysis can confirm that patients with diabetes and hypertension should all be treated with a statin to reduce cholesterol and prevent heart attacks and strokes, as should all patients with diabetes over age forty. But delaying treatment—either to see if the patient can, against the odds, bring their blood pressure down without medications or to conduct a detailed assessment—decreases the number of patients who start treatment, get their blood pressure controlled, and avoid a heart attack or stroke.

3. Prabhdeep Kaur et al., "India Hypertension Control Initiative: Blood Pressure Control Using Drug and Dose-Specific Standard Treatment Protocol at Scale in Punjab and Maharashtra, India, 2022," *Global Heart* 19, no. 1 (March 19, 2024): 30.

4. Andrew E. Moran and Reena Gupta, "Implementation of Global Hearts Hypertension Control Programs in 32 Low- and Middle-Income Countries," *Journal of the American College of Cardiology* 82, no. 19 (November 1, 2023): 1868–1884.

5. Daniel Burka et al., "Keep It Simple: Designing a User-Centred Digital Information System to Support Chronic Disease Management in Low/Middle-Income Countries," *BMJ Health & Care Informatics* 30, no. 1 (January 1, 2023): e100641.

6. Ashish Krishna et al., "Understanding the Role of Staff Nurses in Hypertension Management in Primary Care Facilities in India: A Time-Motion Study," *Preventing Chronic Disease* 20 (May 18, 2023): E39.

7. Barack Obama, "Remarks by President Obama at U.N. Meeting on Ebola" (United Nations Building, New York City, September 25, 2014), https://obamawhitehouse.archives.gov /the-press-office/2014/09/25/remarks-president-obama-un-meeting-ebola.

8. Faisal Shuaib et al., "Ebola Virus Disease Outbreak—Nigeria," 867–872.

9. Tom Frieden, "Former CDC Head on Coronavirus Testing: What Went Wrong and How We Proceed," *USA Today*, April 1, 2020, https://www.usatoday.com/story/opinion/2020/03/31 /former-cdc-head-coronavirus-testing-went-wrong-how-proceed-column/5090097002/. The testing error of the CDC has been widely misunderstood. In an emergency, the CDC's role has always been to rapidly create a limited number of tests for public health laboratories. The CDC did this during the 2009 H1N1 influenza pandemic, disseminating more than a million tests just two weeks after the virus was discovered and providing tests to all states and 140 countries. During COVID, for months the FDA forbade hospitals to create their own versions of these tests, referred to as laboratory-developed tests, for ill patients in hospitals, emergency departments, and outpatient centers. This is the usual way hospitals, which urgently needed tests for critically ill—and worried well—patients coming into emergency departments, get tests done. The Department of Health and Human Services failed to organize and encourage commercial labs to ramp up testing for large numbers of patients in the community, as South Korea did at this time. The CDC's inexcusable error cost lives, but was compounded by the FDA's refusal to allow hospitals to develop their own tests and HHS's failure to mobilize commercial labs. A further misunderstanding has been in the CDC's response to its lab failure, with some observers calling for the United States to have imported the accurate tests being recognized by WHO and used in Germany and elsewhere. The CDC fixed and distributed accurate kits within three weeks of identifying the error; importing, validating and licensing an outside test would have saved little time.

10. New York City Department of Health and Mental Hygiene, "EpiQuery—Syndromic Surveillance Data," accessed March 8, 2025, https://nyc.gov/health/epiquery; Resolve to Save Lives, "Syndromic Surveillance Should Be Explored as an Early Signal for COVID-19," accessed May 6, 2025, https://resolvetosavelives.org/resources/covid-19-in-depth-science -review-march-28-april-3-2020/.

11. "Mayor London Breed Declares Local Emergency to Prepare for Coronavirus," City and County of San Francisco, February 25, 2020, https://www.sf.gov/news/mayor-london -breed-declares-local-emergency-prepare-coronavirus.

12. "Mayor de Blasio Issues State of Emergency," The Official Website of the City of New York, March 13, 2020, https://www.nyc.gov/office-of-the-mayor/news/138-20/mayor-de -blasio-issues-state-emergency.

13. "Timeline: How the Bay Area Has Combated the Coronavirus," *San Francisco Chronicle*, June 19, 2020, https://projects.sfchronicle.com/2020/coronavirus-timeline/.

14. "Mayor de Blasio Issues New Guidance to New Yorkers," The Official Website of the City of New York, March 20, 2020, https://www.nyc.gov/office-of-the-mayor/news/173-20/mayor-de-blasio-issues-new-guidance-new-yorkers.

15. "Transcript: Mayor de Blasio Updates New Yorkers on City's COVID-19 Response," The Official Website of the City of New York, March 9, 2020, https://www.nyc.gov/office-of-the-mayor/news/129-20/transcript-mayor-de-blasio-new-yorkers-city-s-covid-19-response.

16. Jessie Yeung, Adam Renton, Sheena McKenzie, and Meg Wagner, "March 12, 2020 Coronavirus News: 'More and More Restrictions' Are Coming in New York City, Mayor Says," *CNN*, March 12 2020, https://www.cnn.com/world/live-news/coronavirus-outbreak-03-12-20-intl-hnk.

17. "Mayor de Blasio Holds Media Availability on COVID-19," The Official Website of the City of New York, March 15, 2020, https://www.nyc.gov/office-of-the-mayor/news/150-20/mayor-de-blasio-holds-media-availability-covid-19.

18. Chandelis Duster and Paul LeBlanc, "De Blasio Goes to the Gym as Officials Urge Social Distancing to Limit Coronavirus Spread," *CNN*, March 16, 2020, https://www.cnn.com/2020/03/16/politics/bill-de-blasio-gym-coronavirus/index.html.

19. "COVID-19: Data Trends and Totals—NYC Health," New York City Department of Health and Mental Hygiene (2024), accessed March 8, 2025, https://www.nyc.gov/site/doh/covid/covid-19-data-totals.page.

20. "Governor Cuomo Signs the 'New York State on PAUSE' Executive Order," New York State Governor Andrew Cuomo, March 20, 2020, https://www.governor.ny.gov/news/governor-cuomo-signs-new-york-state-pause-executive-order.

21. Farzad Mostashari (@Farzad_MD) on X: "8/ And Continuing to Pursue a Failed Containment Strategy Can Also Delay Making the Hard Decisions Involved in Mitigation. Closing schools Cancelling Events. Telling People to Stay Home. I See No Guidance as to Which Localities Are at This Stage, and What They Should Do," X (Formerly Twitter), March 7, 2020, accessed May 9, 2025, https://twitter.com/Farzad_MD/status/1236401084509368321.

22. Flyvbjerg and Gardner, *How Big Things Get Done*, 115–136.

23. Michael Polanyi, *The Tacit Dimension* (New York: Anchor Books, 1967).

24. Sam Tweed et al., "Increasing Role of Public Health Rapid Response Teams in Infectious Disease Outbreaks," *European Journal of Public Health* 32, Supplement 3 (October 1, 2022).

25. Thomas R. Frieden et al., "7-1-7: An Organising Principle, Target, and Accountability Metric to Make the World Safer From Pandemics," *Lancet* 398, no. 10300 (August 1, 2021): 638–640.

26. Aaron F. Bochner et al., "Implementation of the 7-1-7 Target for Detection, Notification, and Response to Public Health Threats in Five Countries: A Retrospective, Observational Study," *Lancet Global Health* 11, no. 6 (June 1, 2023): e871–879.

27. Although there have been doubts about the health benefits of LPG compared with solid fuels, this primarily reflects inappropriate use of RCTs to assess population-level interventions. See Eric D. McCollum et al., "Liquefied Petroleum Gas or Biomass Cooking and Severe Infant Pneumonia," *New England Journal of Medicine* 390, no. 1 (January 4, 2024): 32–43. This study is an example of using the wrong method to study a public health intervention. Powered to detect a 36 percent decrease in severe pneumonia, the study could have missed a 10–15 percent reduction, which is a plausible impact given the large exposure reductions the study documented and the proven association between exposure and pneumonia (P. L. Kinney et al., "Prenatal and Postnatal Household Air Pollution Exposures and Pneumonia Risk: Evidence from the Ghana Randomized Air Pollution and Health Study," *Chest* 160, no. 5 [2021]: 1634–1644). With an estimated 30 percent of the annual 700,000 child pneumonia deaths attributable to household air pollution, a 10–15 percent reduction would prevent tens of thousands of deaths and millions of cases of pneumonia each year.

   Randomized controlled trials often fail to accurately assess programs that illustrate Rose's prevention paradox: substantial population-wide but limited individual benefit.

28. Adam Fifield, *A Mighty Purpose: How Jim Grant Sold the World on Saving Its Children* (New York: Other Press, 2015); Minta et al., "Progress Toward Measles Elimination—Worldwide, 2000–2022".

29. "Bloomberg Initiative to Reduce Tobacco," Bloomberg Philanthropies, February 14, 2024, accessed March 8, 2025, https://www.bloomberg.org/public-health/reducing-tobacco-use /bloomberg-initiative-to-reduce-tobacco-use/.

30. "Annual Report 2022–2023: Public Health," Bloomberg Philanthropies, July 2, 2024, accessed May 9, 2025, https://web.archive.org/web/20241210213301/https://www.bloom berg.org/annualreport2022/public-health/.

31. Gavin Yamey, "Scaling Up Global Health Interventions: A Proposed Framework for Success," *PLOS Medicine* 8, no. 6 (June 28, 2011): e1001049; Savitha Subramanian et al., "Do We Have the Right Models for Scaling Up Health Services to Achieve the Millennium Development Goals?," *BMC Health Services Research* 11, no. 1 (December 1, 2011): 336; Neil Spicer et al., "'Scaling-Up Is a Craft Not a Science': Catalysing Scale-up of Health Innovations in Ethiopia, India and Nigeria," *Social Science & Medicine* 121 (November 1, 2014): 30–38; Mariam Ashraf et al., "Factors Affecting Successful Scale-Up of Health-Related Pilot Projects," *Journal of the Pakistan Medical Association* 71, no. 2 (October 2020): 524–527; Susan E Bulthuis et al., "Factors Influencing the Scale-Up of Public Health Interventions in Low- and Middle-Income Countries: A Qualitative Systematic Literature Review," *Health Policy and Planning* 35, no. 2 (October 9, 2019): 219–234.

32. Ruth Simmons, Peter Fajans, and Laura Ghiron, *Scaling Up Health Service Delivery: From Pilot Innovations to Policies and Programs* (Geneva, Switzerland: World Health Organization, 2007), https://www.who.int/publications/i/item/9789241563512.

33. David L. Olds, "The Nurse-Family Partnership: An Evidence-Based Preventive Intervention," *Infant Mental Health Journal* 27, no. 1 (January 1, 2006): 5–25.

34. David L. Olds et al., "Long-Term Effects of Home Visitation on Maternal Life Course and Child Abuse and Neglect," *JAMA* 278, no. 8 (August 27, 1997): 637; "Proven Effective Through Extensive Research," *Nurse-Family Partnership*, accessed March 8, 2025, https://www.nursefamilypartnership.org/about/proven-results/.

35. Vijaya Kancherla et al., "Modeling Shows High Potential of Folic Acid-Fortified Salt to Accelerate Global Prevention of Major Neural Tube Defects," *Birth Defects Research* 112, no. 18 (August 1, 2020): 1461–1474.

36. Sumi Mehta et al., "Tackling Air Pollution Starts at Home," *Think Global Health*, February 13, 2013, https://www.thinkglobalhealth.org/article/tackling-air-pollution-starts-home; Perry Hystad et al., "Health Effects of Household Solid Fuel Use: Findings from 11 Countries Within the Prospective Urban and Rural Epidemiology Study," *Environmental Health Perspectives* 127, no. 5 (May 1, 2019).

37. Hugh Sharma Waddington et al., "Impact on Childhood Mortality of Interventions to Improve Drinking Water, Sanitation, and Hygiene (WASH) to Households: Systematic Review and Meta-analysis," *PLOS Medicine* 20, no. 4 (April 20, 2023): e1004215; Obaka Abel Inabo and Noman Arshed, "Impact of Health, Water and Sanitation as Key Drivers of Economic Progress in Nigeria," *African Journal of Science, Technology, Innovation and Development* 11, no. 2 (February 6, 2019): 235–242.

38. World Health Organization, "Global Report on Hypertension."

39. Frances Kateh et al, "Rapid Response to Ebola Outbreaks in Remote Areas—Liberia, July—November 2014," *Morbidity and Mortality Weekly Report* 64, no. 7 (2015): 188–192.

40. Rosling, *Factfulness*, 209.

CHAPTER 7

1. Shankar Vedantam, "The Cassandra Curse," *NPR*, September 17, 2018, https://www.npr.org/transcripts/648781756.

2. Frank I. Luntz. *Words That Work: It's Not What You Say, It's What People Hear* (New York: Hachette Books, 2007).

3. Heather Walker et al., "Forty Years of Slip! Slop! Slap! A Call to Action on Skin Cancer Prevention for Australia," *Public Health Research & Practice* 32, no. 1 (January 1, 2022): 31452117.

4. Jacinda Ardern, "Address to the Nation Announcing Level 4 Lockdown," March 23, 2020, https://www.beehive.govt.nz/speech/prime-minister-covid-19-alert-level-increased.

5. Donald Trump, "Remarks by President Trump in Meeting with African American Leaders," February 27, 2020, https://trumpwhitehouse.archives.gov/briefings-statements/remarks-president-trump-meeting-african-american-leaders/.

6. Charlotte Graham-McLay, "New Zealand Lockdown Releases Charity Spirit as Ardern 'Be Kind' Mantra Kicks In," *Guardian*, July 1, 2020, https://www.theguardian.com/world/2020/apr/22/new-zealand-lockdown-releases-charity-spirit-as-ardern-be-kind-mantra-kicks-in.

7. Bob Cronin, "Trump to Fauci: Why Don't We Let Virus 'Wash Over' Country?," *Newser*, April 12, 2020, https://www.newser.com/story/289449/trump-to-fauci-why-dont-we-let -virus-wash-over-country.html.

8. "Jacinda Ardern Announces Face Mask Mandate for Public Transport, Ubers," *Newshub*, August 24, 2020, https://www.newshub.co.nz/home/new-zealand/2020/08/jacinda-ardern -announces-face-mask-mandate-for-public-transport-ubers.html.

9. Jacinda Ardern, "Pre-Budget Speech to Business New Zealand," May 13, 2021, https://www .beehive.govt.nz/speech/pre-budget-speech-business-new-zealand-1.

10. "Donald Trump Coronavirus Briefing Transcript," April 4, 2020, https://www.rev.com/blog /transcripts/donald-trump-coronavirus-briefing-transcript-april-3-new-cdc-face-mask -recommendations.

11. Saskia Mostert et al., "Excess Mortality Across Countries in the Western World Since the COVID-19 Pandemic: 'Our World in Data' Estimates of January 2020 to December 2022," *BMJ Public Health* 2, no. 1 (May 1, 2024): e000282.

12. U.S. Department of Health and Human Services and U.S. Centers for Disease Control and Prevention, *Crisis Emergency Risk Communication 2014 Edition* (Atlanta, GA: 2014), https:// emergency.cdc.gov/cerc/ppt/cerc_2014edition_Copy.pdf.

13. CDC, "CDC Update on Novel Coronavirus," Transcript for CDC Telebriefing (February 25, 2020), accessed March 8, 2025, https://stacks.cdc.gov/view/cdc/85310/.

14. Isaac Stanley-Becker and Lena H. Sun, "Senior CDC Official Who Met Trump's Wrath for Raising Alarm About Coronavirus to Resign," *Washington Post*, May 7, 2021, https://www .washingtonpost.com/health/2021/05/07/cdc-official-resigns/.

15. Ariel Fridman, Rachel Gershon, and Ayelet Gneezy, "COVID-19 and Vaccine Hesitancy: A Longitudinal Study," *PLOS One* 16, no. 4 (April 16, 2021): e0250123.

16. Kevin C. Davis et al., "Evidence of the Impact of the Tips from Former Smokers Campaign: Results from the Behavioral Risk Factor Surveillance System," *Preventing Chronic Disease* 16 (October 4, 2019): E137; Kevin C. Davis et al., "Association Between Media Doses of the Tips from Former Smokers Campaign and Cessation Behaviors and Intentions to Quit Among Cigarette Smokers, 2012–2015," *Health Education & Behavior* 45, no. 1 (May 12, 2017): 52–60; Kevin Davis et al., "The Impact of the Tips from Former Smokers Campaign on Reducing Cigarette Smoking Relapse," *Journal of Smoking Cessation* 2022 (January 1, 2022): 1–8; Nathan H Mann et al., "The Long-Term Impact of the Tips from Former Smokers Campaign on Calls to 1-800-QUIT-NOW, 2012–2023," *Nicotine & Tobacco Research* 27, no. 2 (2025): 326–332. Studies from controlled trials and observational studies indicate that graphic personal testimonials showing negative health consequences are effective for motivating smoking cessation. See Sarah Durkin, Emily Brennan, and Melanie Wakefield, "Mass Media Campaigns to Promote Smoking Cessation Among Adults: An Integrative Review," *Tobacco Control* 21, no. 2 (February 16, 2012): 127–138; Carlos Sillero-Rejon et al., "Avoidance of Tobacco Health Warnings? An Eye-Tracking Approach," *Addiction* 116, no. 1 (June 7, 2020): 126–138.

17. Jamie Bedson et al., "Community Engagement in Outbreak Response: Lessons from the 2014–2016 Ebola Outbreak in Sierra Leone," *BMJ Global Health* 5, no. 8 (August 1, 2020): e002145.

18. Junko Takeshita et al., "Association of Racial/Ethnic and Gender Concordance Between Patients and Physicians with Patient Experience Ratings," *JAMA Network Open* 3, no. 11 (November 9, 2020): e202458; John E. Snyder et al., "Black Representation in the Primary Care Physician Workforce and Its Association with Population Life Expectancy and Mortality Rates in the US," *JAMA Network Open* 6, no. 4 (April 14, 2023): e236687.

19. Sonia Y. Angell et al., "Cholesterol Control Beyond the Clinic: New York City's Trans Fat Restriction," *Annals of Internal Medicine* 151 (2009): 129–134. Conversations with restaurant chains were instructive. Many purchased a year of oil in advance and argued, reasonably, that they should not be penalized and have to take a large economic loss for the oil they had contracted to buy before the ban was proposed. Dunkin' Donuts pleaded for more time to come up with a new recipe so the sprinkles wouldn't fall off their donuts; we made a donut-hole exemption that gave them more time to phase out trans fats after we figured out how to define a donut for the health code (deep-fried dough, which includes churros). After the regulation passed, McDonald's informed us that they had phased out trans fat in their beloved french fries six months earlier, had done blinded taste tests proving there was no difference, but implored us not to say they had done so; people would believe, falsely, that the fries didn't taste as good.

20. Partnership for Evidence-Based Response to COVID-19 (PERC) "Using Data to Find a Balance," *Resolve to Save Lives*, accessed May 5, 2025, https://resolvetosavelives.org/resources/perc-brief/.

21. "On the Death of His Son, 30 December 1736," *Founders Online*, National Archives, https://founders.archives.gov/documents/Franklin/01-02-02-0025.

22. Mancur Olson, *The Logic of Collective Action: Public Goods and the Theory of Groups* (Cambridge, MA: Harvard University Press, 1965).

23. Frank L. Dewey, "Thomas Jefferson's Law Practice: The Norfolk Anti-Inoculation Riots," *Virginia Magazine of History and Biography* 91, no. 1 (1983): 39–53.

24. Benjamin Franklin, *The Autobiography of Benjamin Franklin* (New Haven, CT: Yale University Press, 1964).

25. "Public Trust in Government: 1958–2023," *U.S. Politics & Policy*, Pew Research Center, January 29, 2024, https://www.pewresearch.org/politics/2023/09/19/public-trust-in-government-1958-2023/.

26. Thomas J. Bollyky et al., "Trust Made the Difference for Democracies in COVID-19," *Lancet* 400, no. 10353 (August 1, 2022): 657.

27. Frank DeStefano and Tom T. Shimabukuro, "The MMR Vaccine and Autism," *Annual Review of Virology* 6, no. 1 (April 15, 2019): 585–600.

28. Di Wang and Zhifei Mao, "A Comparative Study of Public Health and Social Measures of COVID-19 Advocated in Different Countries," *Health Policy* 125, no. 8 (August 1, 2021):

957–971; Wolfgang Stroebe et al., "Politicization of COVID-19 Health-Protective Behaviors in the United States: Longitudinal and Cross-National Evidence," *PLOS One* 16, no. 10 (October 20, 2021): e0256740.

29. Mark Miller, "Focus Group: Vaccine-Hesitant Republicans Want Facts, Not Emotion," De Beaumont Foundation, April 1, 2021, https://debeaumont.org/news/2021/focus-group -vaccines-republicans/; Lulu Garcia-Navarro, "Addressing Vaccine Hesitancy Isn't a One Size Fits All Approach," *Weekend Edition Sunday, NPR*, April 11, 2021, https://www.npr .org/2021/04/11/986203205/addressing-vaccine-hesitancy-isnt-a-one-size-fits-all-approach.

CHAPTER 8

1. Kelly D. Brownell and Thomas R. Frieden, "Ounces of Prevention—the Public Policy Case for Taxes on Sugared Beverages," *New England Journal of Medicine* 360, no. 18 (April 30, 2009): 1805–1808.

2. "Sweet on a Soda Tax?," *Men's Health*, November 2, 2021, https://www.menshealth.com /health/a19524422/sweet-on-a-soda-tax/.

3. David Soll, *Empire of Water: An Environmental and Political History of the New York City Water Supply* (Ithaca, NY: Cornell University Press, 2013).

4. International Union Against Tuberculosis and Lung Disease, "The Union Honours Uruguay's President Tabare Vazquez for His Lasting Contribution to the Global Fight Against Tobacco," *The Union*, December 16, 2020, https://theunion.org/news/the-union-honours -uruguay%E2%80%99s-president-tabare-vazquez-for-his-lasting-contribution-to-the-global -fight-against-tobacco.

5. Danny Hakim, "U.S. Chamber of Commerce Works Globally to Fight Antismoking Measures," *New York Times*, June 30, 2015, https://www.nytimes.com/2015/07/01/business /international/us-chamber-works-globally-to-fight-antismoking-measures.html.

6. Commercial interests have learned this lesson and fund patient groups to advocate for their interests, as occurred during opposition to guidelines to limit inappropriate marketing and prescription of opioid medications. See, for example, *Fueling an Epidemic, Report Two: Exposing the Financial Ties Between Opioid Manufacturers and Third Party Advocacy Groups* (Washington, DC: Committee on Homeland Security and Governmental Affairs, 2018).

7. Tom Farley, *Saving Gotham: A Billionaire Mayor, Activist Doctors, and the Fight for Eight Million Lives* (New York: Norton & Company, 2015).

8. Sarah Stachowiak, *Pathways for Change: 10 Theories to Inform Advocacy and Policy Change Efforts* (Center for Evaluation Innovation and ORS Impact, October 2013), https://evalua tioninnovation.org/wp-content/uploads/2013/11/Pathways-for-Change.pdf.

9. Paulo Serodio et al., "Evaluating Coca-Cola's Attempts to Influence Public Health 'In Their Own Words': Analysis of Coca-Cola Emails with Public Health Academics Leading the Global Energy Balance Network," *Public Health Nutrition* 23, no. 14 (August 3, 2020):

2647–2653; Aditya Kalra et al., "The Philip Morris Files: Part 1: Treaty Blitz—Inside Philip Morris' Campaign to Subvert the Global Anti-Smoking Treaty," Reuters, July 13, 2017.

10. Paul B. Ginsburg and Richard G. Frank, "Pharmaceutical Industry Profits and Research and Development," Brookings, November 17, 2017, https://www.brookings.edu/articles /pharmaceutical-industry-profits-and-research-and-development/.

11. Other medication donation programs have limited impact, and some can be harmful. Donations of expiring, unnecessary, or inappropriate medications, or medications that cannot be used effectively where they are received, do little or no good and may divert the limited national resources needed for more effective programs. See for example, Sally McDonald et al., "Medical Donations Are Not Always Free: An Assessment of Compliance of Medicine and Medical Device Donations with World Health Organization Guidelines (2009–2017)," *International Health* 11, no. 5 (March 21, 2019): 379–402.

12. Kelley Lee and Nicholas Freudenberg, "Public Health Roles in Addressing Commercial Determinants of Health," *Annual Review of Public Health* 43, no. 1 (April 5, 2022): 375–395.

13. Winslow, *The Life of Hermann Biggs*, 40.

14. Sheryl L. Silfen et al., "Increases in Smoking Cessation Interventions After a Feedback and Improvement Initiative Using Electronic Health Records—19 Community Health Centers, New York City, October 2010–March 2012," *Morbidity and Mortality Weekly Report* 63, no. 41 (October 17, 2014): 921–924. Later, when Mayor Bloomberg launched an initiative on climate, the health department designed and received funding for an unprecedented program to track pollutants in the air throughout New York City (Thomas D. Matte et al., "Monitoring Intraurban Spatial Patterns of Multiple Combustion Air Pollutants in New York City: Design and Implementation," *Journal of Exposure Science and Environmental Epidemiology* 23, no. 3 [January 16, 2013]: 223–231). The project used surveillance to see the surprising reality that the worst pollution in the city wasn't from snarled traffic but from the soot belched out by apartment building boilers that used sludge for heating oil. The city then banned these heating oils, substantially improving air quality, reducing asthma, and saving lives.

15. Gabriel T. Rubin, "Congress Eyes Military-Style Budget Carve-Out for Pandemic Prep," *Wall Street Journal*, May 15, 2020, https://www.wsj.com/articles/congress-eyes-military-style -budget-carve-out-for-pandemic-prep-11589535003.

16. Paul Vallely, *Philanthropy: From Aristotle to Zuckerberg* (New York: Bloomsbury Continuum, 2020).

17. Lesley A. Owen and Alastair J. Fischer, "The Cost-Effectiveness of Public Health Interventions Examined by the National Institute for Health and Care Excellence from 2005 to 2018," *Public Health* 169 (April 1, 2019): 151–162.

18. Rebecca Masters et al., "Return on Investment of Public Health Interventions: A Systematic Review," *Journal of Epidemiology and Community Health* 71, no. 8 (March 29, 2017): 827–834; Kirsten Bibbins-Domingo et al., "Projected Effect of Dietary Salt Reductions on Future Cardiovascular Disease," *New England Journal of Medicine* 362, no. 7 (January 20, 2010): 590–599.

19. A. D. Little International Inc., "Public Balance of Smoking in the Czech Republic," Report to Phillip Morris CR (November 28, 2000); Hana Ross, "Critique of the Philip Morris Study of the Cost of Smoking in the Czech Republic," *Nicotine & Tobacco Research* 6, no. 1 (2004): 181–189.

20. Rose, *Preventive Medicine*, 38.

21. M. R. Gasner et al., "The Use of Legal Action in New York City to Ensure Treatment of Tuberculosis," *New England Journal of Medicine* 340, no. 5 (February 4, 1999): 359–366.

22. Gabriel Feldman et al., "Detention Until Cure as a Last Resort: New York City's Experience With Involuntary In-Hospital Civil Detention of Persistently Nonadherent Tuberculosis Patients," *Seminars in Respiratory and Critical Care Medicine* 18, no. 05 (September 1, 1997): 493–501.

23. Sara Hersey et al., "Ebola Virus Disease—Sierra Leone and Guinea, August 2015," *Morbidity and Mortality Weekly Report* 64, no. 35 (September 11, 2015): 981–984; Sakoba Keita, *My Fight Against Ebola in the Republic of Guinea* (Paris: L'Harmattan, 2022).

24. Geoff Manaugh and Nicola Twilley, *Until Proven Safe: The History and Future of Quarantine* (London: Pan Macmillan, 2021).

25. Resolve to Save Lives, "Alert-Level Systems for COVID-19—Prevent Epidemics," accessed May 6, 2025, https://resolvetosavelives.org/resources/covid-19-risk-alert-levels/.

26. Particularly when others are not masked, vulnerable people are likely much better protected with a well-fitting N95 or KN95 mask. See, for example, Andrew P. Collins et al., "N95 Respirator and Surgical Mask Effectiveness Against Respiratory Viral Illnesses in the Healthcare Setting: A Systematic Review and Meta-Analysis," *Journal of the American College of Emergency Physicians Open* 2, no. 5 (October 1, 2021): e12582.

27. Lidia Kuznetsova, Giorgio Cortassa, and Antoni Trilla, "Effectiveness of Mandatory and Incentive-Based Routine Childhood Immunization Programs in Europe: A Systematic Review of the Literature," *Vaccines* 9, no. 10 (October 13, 2021): 1173; Varun K. Phadke et al., "Association Between Vaccine Refusal and Vaccine-Preventable Diseases in the United States," *JAMA* 315, no. 11 (March 15, 2016): 1149.

28. Employer-based COVID vaccination mandates may be more defensible, in part because they reduce absenteeism and workplace disruption, protect vulnerable staff and clients, and reduce health insurance costs.

29. Chester Bernard, *Functions of the Executive* (Cambridge, MA: Harvard University Press, 1938).

30. Thomas R. Frieden and Jeffrey P. Koplan, "Stronger National Public Health Institutes for Global Health," *Lancet* 376, no. 9754 (November 1, 2010): 1721–1722.

31. John Coggon, *The Nanny State Debate: A Place Where Words Don't Do Justice* (London: Faculty of Public Health, 2018), https://www.fph.org.uk/media/1972/fph-nannystatedebate-report-final.pdf.

32. Daniel M. Fox, "Social Policy and City Politics: Tuberculosis Reporting in New York, 1889–1900," *Bulletin of the History of Medicine* 49, no. 2 (Summer 1975): 169–175.

33. Scott Kaplan et al., "Evaluation of Changes in Prices and Purchases Following Implementation of Sugar-Sweetened Beverage Taxes Across the US," *JAMA Health Forum* 5, no. 1 (January 5, 2024): e234737.

34. James Flynn, "Soda Taxes, Consumption, and Health Outcomes for High School Students," *Economics Letters* 234 (December 28, 2023): 111507; Deborah Rohm Young et al., "City-Level Sugar-Sweetened Beverage Taxes and Youth Body Mass Index Percentile," *JAMA Network Open* 7, no. 7 (July 31, 2024): e2424822.

35. Ryan M. Kane and Vasanti S. Malik, "Understanding Beverage Taxation: Perspective on the Philadelphia Beverage Tax's Novel Approach," *Journal of Public Health Research* 8, no. 1 (March 11, 2019): jphr.2019.1466.

36. Scott L. Greer et al., "Policy, Politics and Public Health," *European Journal of Public Health* 27, Supplement 4 (October 1, 2017): 40–43; Heather Marquette, "Political Will: What It Is, Why It Matters for Extractives, and How on Earth Do You Find It?," Columbia Center on Sustainable Investment, February 20, 2020, https://ccsi.columbia.edu/news/political-will-what-it-why-it-matters-extractives-and-how-earth-do-you-find-it; David Pedley, "Understanding Change as Politics Not Political Will," Foreign, Commonwealth & Development Office, July 17, 2024, https://www.gov.uk/government/publications/understanding-change-as-politics-not-political-will/understanding-change-as-politics-not-political-will.

CHAPTER 9

1. "The Pandemic's True Death Toll," *Economist*, October 25, 2022, https://www.economist.com/graphic-detail/coronavirus-excess-deaths-estimates; Benjamin Bowe, Yan Xie, and Ziyad Al-Aly, "Postacute Sequelae of COVID-19 at 2 Years," *Nature Medicine (Print)* 29, no. 9 (August 21, 2023): 2347–2357; Terrie Walmsley et al., "Macroeconomic Consequences of the COVID-19 Pandemic," *Economic Modelling* 120 (March 1, 2023): 106147.

2. Matt Craven et al., "Not the Last Pandemic: Investing Now to Reimagine Public-Health Systems," McKinsey & Company, May 21, 2021, https://www.mckinsey.com/industries/public-sector/our-insights/not-the-last-pandemic-investing-now-to-reimagine-public-health-systems.

3. Scott Hershberger, "The 1918 Flu Faded in Our Collective Memory: We Might 'Forget' the Coronavirus, Too," *Scientific American*, August 13, 2020, https://www.scientificamerican.com/article/the-1918-flu-faded-in-our-collective-memory-we-might-forget-the-coronavirus-too/.

4. Thomas R. Frieden et al., "Tuberculosis in New York City—Turning the Tide," *New England Journal of Medicine* 333, no. 4 (July 27, 1995): 229–233; New York City Department of Health and Mental Hygiene, *Bureau of Tuberculosis Control Annual Summary* (Long Island City, New York, 2024), https://www.nyc.gov/assets/doh/downloads/pdf/tb/tuberculosis-in-new-york-city-2023-annual-report.pdf.

5. Michelle Rozo and Gigi Kwik Grönvall, "The Reemergent 1977 H1N1 Strain and the Gain-of-Function Debate," *MBio* 6, no. 4 (September 1, 2015).

6. House of Commons, *Report of the Investigation into the Cause of the 1978 Birmingham Smallpox Occurrence* (London: Her Majesty's Stationery Office, July 22, 1980), https://assets.publishing.service.gov.uk/government/uploads/system/uploads/attachment_data/file/228654/0668.pdf.pdf.

7. Dennis Normile, "Mounting Lab Accidents Raise SARS Fears," *Science* 304, no. 5671 (April 30, 2004): 659–661.

8. Richard Fausset and Donald G. McNeil Jr., "After Lapses, C.D.C. Admits a Lax Culture at Labs," *New York Times*, July 14, 2014, https://www.nytimes.com/2014/07/14/us/after-lapses-cdc-admits-a-lax-culture-at-labs.html; Denise Grady and Donald G. McNeil Jr., "Ebola Sample Is Mishandled at C.D.C. Lab in Latest Error," *New York Times*, December 24, 2014, https://www.nytimes.com/2014/12/25/health/cdc-ebola-error-in-lab-may-have-exposed-technician-to-virus.html; U.S. Centers for Disease Control and Prevention, *Report on the Potential Exposure to Anthrax* (July 11, 2014), https://www.cdc.gov/labs/pdf/Final_Anthrax_Report.pdf; Richard Harris, "Smallpox Virus Found in Unsecured NIH Lab," *NPR*, July 8, 2014, https://www.npr.org/sections/health-shots/2014/07/08/329847454/smallpox-virus-found-in-unsecured-nih-freezer.

9. Independent Task Force on Research with Pandemic Risks, *A Framework for Tomorrow's Pathogen Research* (Chicago: Bulletin of the Atomic Scientists, 2024), https://thebulletin.org/wp-content/uploads/2024/02/Pathogens-Project_A-Framework-for-Tomorrows-Pathogen-Research_Final-Report-2024.pdf.

10. National Science Advisory Board for Biosecurity, *Recommendations for the Evaluation and Oversight of Proposed Gain-of-Function Research* (May 2016), https://osp.od.nih.gov/wp-content/uploads/2016/06/NSABB_Final_Report_Recommendations_Evaluation_Oversight_Proposed_Gain_of_Function_Research.pdf.

11. Serge Morand and Claire Lajaunie, "Outbreaks of Vector-Borne and Zoonotic Diseases Are Associated with Changes in Forest Cover and Oil Palm Expansion at Global Scale," *Frontiers in Veterinary Science* 8 (March 24, 2021): 661063.

12. Jesús Olivero et al., "Recent Loss of Closed Forests Is Associated with Ebola Virus Disease Outbreaks," *Scientific Reports* 7, no. 1 (October 30, 2017): 14291.

13. Neil M. Vora et al., "Interventions to Reduce Risk for Pathogen Spillover and Early Disease Spread to Prevent Outbreaks, Epidemics, and Pandemics," *Emerging Infectious Diseases* 29, no. 3 (March 1, 2023): 1–9.

14. Daniel C. Nepstad et al., "Slowing Amazon Deforestation Through Public Policy and Interventions in Beef and Soy Supply Chains," *Science* 344, no. 6188 (June 6, 2014): 1118–1123.

15. Vanda Felbab-Brown, "Reopening the World: To Prevent Zoogenic Pandemics, Regulate Wildlife Trade and Food Production," Brookings, June 16, 2020, https://www.brookings

.edu/articles/reopening-the-world-to-prevent-zoogenic-pandemics-regulate-wildlife-trade
-and-food-production/.

16. Amanda McClelland and Thomas R. Frieden, "Ongoing Cholera Pandemic Shows Need to Go Back to Basics for Healthier Today and Safer Tomorrow," *CNN*, June 1, 2023, https://edition.cnn.com/2023/06/01/health/ongoing-cholera-pandemic.

17. Steven Johnson, *The Ghost Map: The Story of London's Most Terrifying Epidemic—and How It Changed Science, Cities, and the Modern World* (New York: Riverhead Books, 2006); Nancy Mandelker Frieden, *Russian Physicians in an Era of Reform and Revolution* (Princeton, NJ: Princeton University Press, 1981), 158–159.

18. Deepak Balasubramanian et al., "Cholera Dynamics: Lessons from an Epidemic," *Journal of Medical Microbiology* 70, no. 2 (February 1, 2021).

19. *Vital Statistics. Twelfth Census of the United States, Taken in the Year 1900*, vol. IV, part II, *Statistics of Deaths* (Washington, DC: United States Census Office, 1902); U.S. Centers for Disease Control and Prevention, "CDC Wonder Online Database: Multiple Causes of Death 2018–2023," accessed March 8, 2025, http://wonder.cdc.gov/mcd.html.

20. Mensah et al., "Decline in Cardiovascular Mortality."

21. Gawande, *Checklist Manifesto*.

22. Brenda Reiss-Brennan et al., "Association of Integrated Team-Based Care with Health Care Quality, Utilization, and Cost," *JAMA* 316, no. 8 (August 23, 2016): 826; Maximilian J. Pany et al., "Provider Teams Outperform Solo Providers in Managing Chronic Diseases and Could Improve the Value of Care," *Health Affairs* 40, no. 3 (March 1, 2021): 435–444.

23. Julian Tudor Hart, "The Inverse Care Law," *Lancet* 297, no. 7696 (February 1, 1971): 405–412.

24. Juan Rafael Vargas and Jorine Muiser, "Promoting Universal Financial Protection: A Policy Analysis of Universal Health Coverage in Costa Rica (1940–2000)," *Health Research Policy and Systems* 11, no. 1 (August 21, 2013): 28.

25. Mensah et al., "Decline in Cardiovascular Mortality."

26. Farapti Farapti et al., "Community-Level Dietary Intake of Sodium, Potassium, and Sodium-to-Potassium Ratio as a Global Public Health Problem: A Systematic Review and Meta-Analysis," *F1000Research* 11 (September 30, 2024): 953.

27. Neal et al., "Effect of Salt Substitution on Cardiovascular Events and Death."

28. "FDA Issues Voluntary Sodium Reduction Targets"; Jacobson, *Salt Wars*.

29. Nicole Ide et al., "Priority Actions to Advance Population Sodium Reduction," *Nutrients* 12, no. 9 (August 22, 2020): 2543.

30. Sarah Pickersgill et al., "Modeling Global 80-80-80 Blood Pressure Targets and Cardiovascular Outcomes," *Nature Medicine* 28, no. 8 (July 18, 2022): 1693–1699. Data also drawn

from Institute for Health Metrics and Evaluation (IHME), Global Burden of Disease (2024), with processing by Our World in Data, "Number of Deaths from Hypertension," Global Burden of Disease—Risk Factors, retrieved March 23, 2025, from https://ourworldindata.org /grapher/deaths-due-to-high-blood-pressure. Remarkably, this estimate is limited to improving treatment of hypertension. By improving both treatment and prevention, an even faster, deeper decrease in cardiovascular disease deaths is possible.

CHAPTER 10

1. G. Mancia, "Scipione Riva-Rocci," *Clinical Cardiology* 20, no. 5 (May 1, 1997): 503–504. Riva-Rocci refused to patent his invention, freely shared it with others, and emphasized that blood pressure monitors could be constructed from inexpensive and readily available materials.

2. Prospective Studies Collaboration, "Age-Specific Relevance of Usual Blood Pressure to Vascular Mortality: A Meta-Analysis of Individual Data for One Million Adults in 61 Prospective Studies," *Lancet* 360, no. 9349 (December 1, 2002): 1903–1913.

3. Defined as having blood pressure above 115/70 or being on antihypertensive medications. Calculated using data from the CDC's *National Health and Nutrition Examination Survey (NHANES)* (2017–March 2020), unpublished.

4. E. Murat Tuzcu et al., "High Prevalence of Coronary Atherosclerosis in Asymptomatic Teenagers and Young Adults," *Circulation* 103, no. 22 (June 5, 2001): 2705–2710.

5. Peter Attia and Bill Gifford, *Outlive: The Science and Art of Longevity* (New York: Harmony Books, 2023). LDL cholesterol has been thought of as the unhealthy cholesterol and HDL as healthy. Studies at CDC and elsewhere show that LDL and HDL consist of hundreds of molecules, including some cardioprotective LDL molecules and some harmful HDL molecules. Understanding of lipids is evolving rapidly; as of 2025, the primary indicators to track unhealthy cholesterol are ApoB and LDL-C. New lipid tests will become available in the coming years. For more on ApoB and LDL-C, see for example Tamara Glavinovic et al., "Physiological Bases for the Superiority of Apolipoprotein B Over Low-Density Lipoprotein Cholesterol and Non–High-Density Lipoprotein Cholesterol as a Marker of Cardiovascular Risk," *Journal of the American Heart Association* 11, no. 20 (October 18, 2022): e025858.

6. Joshua C. Denny and Francis S. Collins, "Precision Medicine in 2030—Seven Ways to Transform Healthcare," *Cell* 184, no. 6 (March 1, 2021): 1415–1419.

7. "Microbiome," National Institute of Environmental Health Sciences, March 22, 2024, accessed March 8, 2025, https://www.niehs.nih.gov/health/topics/science/microbiome; Andrew P. Shoubridge et al., "The Gut Microbiome and Mental Health: Advances in Research and Emerging Priorities," *Molecular Psychiatry* 27, no. 4 (March 2, 2022): 1908–1919.

8. Olga Castaner et al., "The Gut Microbiome Profile in Obesity: A Systematic Review," *International Journal of Endocrinology* 2018 (January 1, 2018): 1–9.

9. "Microbiome," NIEHS; Shoubridge et al., "The Gut Microbiome and Mental Health"; Jens Puschhof and Eran Elinav, "Human Microbiome Research: Growing Pains and Future Promises," *PLOS Biology* 21, no. 3 (March 17, 2023): e3002053.

10. Tarini Shankar Ghosh and Ana Maria Valdes, "Evidence for Clinical Interventions Targeting the Gut Microbiome in Cardiometabolic Disease," *BMJ* 383 (October 9, 2023): e075180. The topic of ultraprocessed foods is complex. Definitions of such foods differ, and some ultraprocessed foods may be healthier than some unprocessed foods. We'll learn much more in the coming years.

11. Michael Lewis, "Don't Eat Fortune's Cookie," Princeton University's 2012 Baccalaureate Remarks, June 3, 2012, https://www.princeton.edu/news/2012/06/03/princeton -universitys-2012-baccalaureate-remarks.

12. National Academies of Sciences, *Public Health Consequences of E-Cigarettes* (Washington, DC: National Academies Press, 2018).

13. Josef Hamoud et al., "A Systematic Review Investigating the Impact of Dual Use of E-Cigarettes and Conventional Cigarettes on Smoking Cessation," *ERJ Open Research* (2024): 00902-2024, https://doi.org/10.1183/23120541.00902-2024.

14. SPRINT, "A Randomized Trial of Intensive Versus Standard Blood-Pressure Control"; Jeremiah Stamler et al., "Low Risk-Factor Profile and Long-Term Cardiovascular and Noncardiovascular Mortality and Life Expectancy," *JAMA* 282, no. 21 (December 1, 1999): 2012–2018.

15. Brian A. Ference et al., "Low-Density Lipoproteins Cause Atherosclerotic Cardiovascular Disease. 1. Evidence from Genetic, Epidemiologic, and Clinical Studies. A Consensus Statement from the European Atherosclerosis Society Consensus Panel," *European Heart Journal* 38, no. 32 (March 9, 2017): 2459–2472; Attia and Gifford, *Outlive*; Marc S. Sabatine et al., "Efficacy and Safety of Further Lowering of Low-Density Lipoprotein Cholesterol in Patients Starting with Very Low Levels," *JAMA Cardiology* 3, no. 9 (August 1, 2018): 823–828.

16. Bente Klarlund Pedersen and Bengt Saltin, "Exercise as Medicine—Evidence for Prescribing Exercise as Therapy in 26 Different Chronic Diseases," *Scandinavian Journal of Medicine & Science in Sports* 25, no. S3 (November 25, 2015): 1–72. Pet ownership in general, and dog ownership in particular, has been associated with improved outcomes; this may be the result of increased physical activity from dog-walking.

17. Kelly R. Tan et al., "Neural Bases for Addictive Properties of Benzodiazepines," *Nature* 463, no. 7282 (February 1, 2010): 769–774; Charles P. O'Brien, "Benzodiazepine Use, Abuse, and Dependence," *Journal of Clinical Psychiatry* 66, Supplement 2 (2005): 28–33; Susan Golombok, Parimala Moodley, and Malcolm Lader, "Cognitive Impairment in Long-Term Benzodiazepine Users," *Psychological Medicine* 18, no. 2 (May 1, 1988): 365–374; Matthew E. Hirschtritt, Mark Olfson, and Kurt Kroenke, "Balancing the Risks and Benefits of Benzodiazepines," *JAMA* 325, no. 4 (January 13, 2021): 347–348.

18. Yuan Ma et al., "24-Hour Urinary Sodium and Potassium Excretion and Cardiovascular Risk," *New England Journal of Medicine* 386, no. 3 (January 20, 2022): 252–263; Aburto et

al., "Effect of Increased Potassium Intake on Cardiovascular Risk Factors and Disease"; Zhang et al., "Association Between Usual Sodium and Potassium Intake and Blood Pressure and Hypertension." Although not directly proven to increase longevity, studies have shown that lower sodium and higher potassium intake reduce blood pressure, heart attacks, and strokes.

19. International Agency for Research on Cancer, *Red Meat and Processed Meat* (Lyon, France: IARC, 2018).

20. Ahmed S. BaHammam and Abdulrouf Pirzada, "Timing Matters: The Interplay Between Early Mealtime, Circadian Rhythms, Gene Expression, Circadian Hormones, and Metabolism—A Narrative Review," *Clocks & Sleep* 5, no. 3 (September 6, 2023): 507–535; Marie-Pierre St-Onge et al., "Meal Timing and Frequency: Implications for Cardiovascular Disease Prevention: A Scientific Statement From the American Heart Association," *Circulation* 135, no. 9 (February 28, 2017): e96–121.

21. Yan Zheng et al., "Association of Changes in Red Meat Consumption with Total and Cause Specific Mortality Among US Women and Men: Two Prospective Cohort Studies," *BMJ* (June 12, 2019): 12110. Some authorities would place reducing red meat consumption in the "strong scientific evidence" category. Health effects of reducing unprocessed red meat consumption will depend on what it is replaced with, whether protein and other nutrient needs are met, and the baseline and new level of unprocessed red meat consumption. In any case, reducing red meat consumption has substantial environmental benefits.

22. Ruth E. Patterson and Dorothy D. Sears, "Metabolic Effects of Intermittent Fasting," *Annual Review of Nutrition* 37, no. 1 (August 21, 2017): 371–393; Rafael De Cabo and Mark P. Mattson, "Effects of Intermittent Fasting on Health, Aging, and Disease," *New England Journal of Medicine* 381, no. 26 (December 25, 2019): 2541–2551.

23. Sina Naghshi et al., "Dietary Intake of Total, Animal, and Plant Proteins and Risk of All Cause, Cardiovascular, and Cancer Mortality: Systematic Review and Dose-Response Meta-Analysis of Prospective Cohort Studies," *BMJ* 370 (July 22, 2020): m2412; Mingyang Song et al., "Association of Animal and Plant Protein Intake with All-Cause and Cause-Specific Mortality," *JAMA Internal Medicine* 176, no. 10 (October 1, 2016): 1453–1463; Nuno Mendonça et al., "Low Protein Intake, Physical Activity, and Physical Function in European and North American Community-dwelling Older Adults: A Pooled Analysis of Four Longitudinal Aging Cohorts," *American Journal of Clinical Nutrition* 114, no. 1 (July 1, 2021): 29–41.

24. Séverine Sabia et al., "Association of Sleep Duration in Middle and Old Age with Incidence of Dementia," *Nature Communications* 12, no. 1 (April 20, 2021): 2289.

25. Jayandra J. Himali et al., "Association Between Slow-Wave Sleep Loss and Incident Dementia," *JAMA Neurology* 80, no. 12 (December 1, 2023): 1326–1333.

26. Joshua R. Ehrlich et al., "Addition of Vision Impairment to a Life-Course Model of Potentially Modifiable Dementia Risk Factors in the US," *JAMA Neurology* 79, no. 6 (June 1, 2022): 623–626; Frank R. Lin et al., "Hearing Loss and Cognitive Decline in Older Adults," *JAMA Internal Medicine* 173, no. 4 (February 25, 2013): 293–299.

27. Fergus I. M. Craik, Ellen Bialystok, and Morris Freedman, "Delaying the Onset of Alzheimer Disease: Bilingualism as a Form of Cognitive Reserve," *Neurology* 75, no. 19 (November 9, 2010): 1726–1729; Ahmed Arafa et al., "Playing a Musical Instrument and the Risk of Dementia Among Older Adults: A Systematic Review and Meta-analysis of Prospective Cohort Studies," *BMC Neurology* 22, no. 1 (October 27, 2022): 35.

28. Jieyu Zhang et al., "A Meta-Analysis of Cohort Studies: Traumatic Brain Injury and Risk of Alzheimer's Disease," *PLOS One* 16, no. 6 (June 22, 2021): e0253206.

29. Fan Wang et al., "A Systematic Review and Meta-Analysis of 90 Cohort Studies of Social Isolation, Loneliness and Mortality," *Nature Human Behaviour* 7, no. 8 (June 19, 2023): 1307–1319. Although social isolation correlates with worse health outcomes, this association may not be causal. Also, there is limited evidence that interventions to reduce social isolation are effective in the long term or that these interventions increase disability-free longevity. There are studies from Finland that suggest that sauna bathing at least four days per week is associated with longer, dementia-free survival (see, e.g., Tanjaniina Laukkanen et al., "Sauna Bathing Is Inversely Associated With Dementia and Alzheimer's Disease in Middle-aged Finnish Men," *Age and Ageing* 46, no. 2 [December 8, 2016]: 245–249); this finding may not be broadly applicable. Breathing exercises have been associated with lower blood pressures, but no trial has documented either long-term adherence or long-term health benefits.

30. H. J. Naurath et al., "Effects of Vitamin B12, Folate, and Vitamin B6 Supplements in Elderly People with Normal Serum Vitamin Concentrations," *Lancet* 346, no. 8967 (July 1, 1995): 85–89; Ralph Green et al., "Vitamin B12 Deficiency," *Nature Reviews Disease Primers* 3, no. 1 (June 29, 2017): 17040.

31. May A. Beydoun et al., "Clinical and Bacterial Markers of Periodontitis and Their Association with Incident All-Cause and Alzheimer's Disease Dementia in a Large National Survey," *Journal of Alzheimer's Disease* 75, no. 1 (May 5, 2020): 157–172.

32. Ralph Green, "Vitamin B12 Deficiency from the Perspective of a Practicing Hematologist," *Blood* 129, no. 19 (May 11, 2017): 2603–2611.

33. William Shakespeare, *As You Like It,* act 2, scene 7.

34. Aina Najwa Mohd Khairuddin et al., "Impact of Dental Visiting Patterns on Oral Health: A Systematic Review of Longitudinal Studies," *BDJ Open* 10, no. 18 (March 6, 2024); Matthew J. Burton et al., "The Lancet Global Health Commission on Global Eye Health: Vision Beyond 2020," *Lancet Global Health* 9, no. 4 (February 16, 2021): e489–e551.

35. National Academies of Sciences, Engineering, and Medicine, *Myopia: Causes, Prevention, and Treatment of an Increasingly Common Disease* (Washington, DC: National Academies Press, 2024).

36. "Noise as a Public Health Hazard," American Public Health Association, October 26, 2021, https://www.apha.org/Policies-and-Advocacy/Public-Health-Policy-Statements/Policy -Database/2022/01/07/Noise-as-a-Public-Health-Hazard.

37. Jeremiah Stamler, "The INTERSALT Study: Background, Methods, Findings, and Implications," *American Journal of Clinical Nutrition* 65, no. 2 (February 1, 1997): 626S–642S; Kazem Rahimi, "Mounting Evidence in Favour of the Lower, the Better Blood Pressure Paradigm," *Lancet*, 404, no. 10449 (July 20, 2024): 216–217.

38. Lilian Jans-Beken et al., "Gratitude and Health: An Updated Review," *Journal of Positive Psychology* 15, no. 6 (August 6, 2019): 743–782; Sensen Zhang, Yulun Tang, and Shaohong Yong, "The Influence of Gratitude on Pre-Service Teachers' Career Goal Self-Efficacy: Chained Intermediary Analysis of Meaning in Life and Career Calling," *Frontiers in Psychology* 13 (July 28, 2022): 843276.

39. Benjamin Gardner, Phillippa Lally, and Jane Wardle, "Making Health Habitual: The Psychology of 'Habit-Formation' and General Practice," *British Journal of General Practice* 62, no. 605 (December 1, 2012): 664–666.

40. Hayami K. Koga et al., "Optimism, Lifestyle, and Longevity in a Racially Diverse Cohort of Women," *Journal of the American Geriatrics Society* 70, no. 10 (June 8, 2022): 2793–2804; Lewina O. Lee et al., "Optimism Is Associated with Exceptional Longevity in Two Epidemiologic Cohorts of Men and Women," *Proceedings of the National Academy of Sciences of the United States of America* 116, no. 37 (August 26, 2019): 18357–18362; Eric S. Kim et al., "Optimism and Cause-Specific Mortality: A Prospective Cohort Study," *American Journal of Epidemiology* 185, no. 1 (December 7, 2016): 21–29.

41. Jacquelyn Jacobs et al., "Impact of a Multi-disciplinary Team-Based Care Model for Patients Living with Diabetes on Health Outcomes: A Mixed-Methods Study," *BMC Health Services Research* 24, no. 1 (June 18, 2024): 746; Timothy W. Levengood et al., "Team-Based Care to Improve Diabetes Management: A Community Guide Meta-Analysis," *American Journal of Preventive Medicine* 57, no. 1 (July 1, 2019): e17–26; Pany et al., "Provider Teams Outperform Solo Providers"; "Community Health Workers," The Community Guide, September 20, 2017, accessed January 12, 2025, https://web.archive.org/web/20250112202532 /https://www.thecommunityguide.org/pages/community-health-workers.html.

42. "Information for Consumers," United States Preventive Services Taskforce, 2024, accessed March 25, 2025, https://www.uspreventiveservicestaskforce.org/uspstf/recommendation -topics/information-for-consumers; "NICE Guidance," National Institute for Health and Care Excellence (NICE), July 24, 2024, accessed March 25, 2025 https://www.nice.org .uk/guidance.

43. Veterans Administration Cooperative Study Group on Antihypertensive Agents, "Effects of Treatment on Morbidity in Hypertension," *JAMA* 202, no. 11 (December 11, 1967): 1028; Veterans Administration Cooperative Study Group on Antihypertensive Agents, "Effects of Treatment on Morbidity in Hypertension," *JAMA* 213, no. 7 (August 17, 1970): 1143.

44. SPRINT, "A Randomized Trial of Intensive Versus Standard Blood-Pressure Control."

45. Ference et al., "Low-Density Lipoproteins Cause Atherosclerotic Cardiovascular Disease"; Attia and Gifford, *Outlive*; Sabatine et al., "Efficacy and Safety of Further Lowering of Low-Density Lipoprotein Cholesterol." See also endnote 5 in this chapter.

46. Pedersen and Saltin, "Exercise as Medicine."

47. Caoimhe Twohig-Bennett and Andy Jones, "The Health Benefits of the Great Outdoors: A Systematic Review and Meta-Analysis of Greenspace Exposure and Health Outcomes," *Environmental Research* 166 (October 1, 2018): 628–637.

48. N. J. Aburto et al., "Effect of Lower Sodium Intake on Health: Systematic Review and Meta-Analyses," *BMJ* 346, no. 3 (April 3, 2013): f1326; Joanne L. Slavin and Beate Lloyd, "Health Benefits of Fruits and Vegetables," *Advances in Nutrition* 3, no. 4 (July 1, 2012): 506–516; Wenming Shi et al., "Red Meat Consumption, Cardiovascular Diseases, and Diabetes: A Systematic Review and Meta-Analysis," *European Heart Journal* 44, no. 28 (June 2, 2023): 2626–2635; Zheng et al., "Association of Changes in Red Meat Consumption"; International Agency for Research on Cancer, *Red Meat and Processed Meat*.

49. Ma et al., "24-Hour Urinary Sodium and Potassium Excretion and Cardiovascular Risk"; Aburto et al., "Effect of Increased Potassium Intake on Cardiovascular Risk Factors and Disease."

50. Zefeng Zhang et al., "Association Between Usual Sodium and Potassium Intake and Blood Pressure and Hypertension Among U.S. Adults: NHANES 2005–2010," *PLOS One* 8, no. 10 (October 10, 2013): e75289.

51. BaHammam and Pirzada, "Timing Matters"; St-Onge et al., "Meal Timing and Frequency."

52. Bo-Huei Huang et al., "Influence of Poor Sleep on Cardiovascular Disease-Free Life Expectancy: A Multi-Resource-Based Population Cohort Study," *BMC Medicine* 21, no. 1 (March 2, 2023): 75; Kristen L Knutson et al., "The Metabolic Consequences of Sleep Deprivation," *Sleep Medicine Reviews* 11, no. 3 (June 1, 2007): 163–178; Christina Antza et al., "The Links Between Sleep Duration, Obesity and Type 2 Diabetes Mellitus," *Journal of Endocrinology* 252, no. 2 (2022): 125–141.

53. Carla De Pasquale et al., "Sleep Hygiene—What Do We Mean? A Bibliographic Review," *Sleep Medicine Reviews* (April 1, 2024): 101930; Leah A. Irish et al., "The Role of Sleep Hygiene in Promoting Public Health: A Review of Empirical Evidence," *Sleep Medicine Reviews* 22 (August 1, 2015): 23–36.

54. Lauren Hale and Stanford Guan, "Screen Time and Sleep Among School-aged Children and Adolescents: A Systematic Literature Review," *Sleep Medicine Reviews* 21 (June 1, 2015): 50–58; Tobias Stächele et al., "Effects of a 6-Week Internet-Based Stress Management Program on Perceived Stress, Subjective Coping Skills, and Sleep Quality," *Frontiers in Psychiatry* 11 (May 25, 2020). There is some evidence that reducing stress increases longevity. The problem with studies such as these is the danger of what is known as residual confounding—that one or more factors cause both greater stress and shorter lives, an effect that statistical tests may not adequately correct.

55. Prabhat Jha and Richard Peto, "Global Effects of Smoking, of Quitting, and of Taxing Tobacco," *New England Journal of Medicine* 370, no. 1 (January 2, 2014): 60–68.

56. David R. Arday et al., "Smoking and Functional Status Among Medicare Managed Care Enrollees," *American Journal of Preventive Medicine* 24, no. 3 (April 1, 2003): 234–241; Neil Mehta and Mikko Myrskylä, "The Population Health Benefits of a Healthy Lifestyle: Life Expectancy Increased and Onset of Disability Delayed," *Health Affairs* 36, no. 8 (August 1, 2017): 1495–1502.

57. US Department of Health and Human Services, *Smoking Cessation: A Report of the Surgeon General*, chapter 4, "The Health Benefits of Smoking Cessation," Washington, DC: U.S. Public Health Service, Office of the Surgeon General; National Center for Chronic Disease Prevention and Health Promotion, Office on Smoking and Health, 2020, https://www.ncbi.nlm.nih.gov/books/NBK555590/. For resources to quit smoking, see "How to Quit Smoking," Centers for Disease Control and Prevention, September 15, 2023, accessed March 8, 2025, https://www.cdc.gov/tobacco/campaign/tips/quit-smoking/index.html; "Tools & Tips," National Institutes of Health, 2024, accessed March 8, 2025, https://smokefree.gov/.

58. E. Prescott, "Importance of Light Smoking and Inhalation Habits on Risk of Myocardial Infarction and All-Cause Mortality: A 22 Year Follow-Up of 12,149 Men and Women in the Copenhagen City Heart Study," *Journal of Epidemiology and Community Health* 56, no. 9 (September 1, 2002): 702–706.

59. Rose, *Preventive Medicine*, 118.

60. Binge drinking is defined as four or more drinks for women and five or more drinks for men on one occasion. Drinking on average more than one or two drinks a day is considered heavy drinking.

61. Scott E. Hadland et al., "Association of Pharmaceutical Industry Marketing of Opioid Products with Mortality from Opioid-Related Overdoses," *JAMA Network Open* 2, no. 1 (January 18, 2019): e186007; Svetlana Beilfuss and Sebastian Linde, "Pharmaceutical Opioid Marketing and Physician Prescribing Behavior," *Health Economics* 30, no. 12 (September 25, 2021): 3159–3185.

62. Deborah Dowell et al., "CDC Clinical Practice Guideline for Prescribing Opioids for Pain—United States, 2022," *MMWR Recommendations and Reports* 71, no. 3 (November 4, 2022): 1–95.

63. Tan et al., "Neural Bases for Addictive Properties of Benzodiazepines"; O'Brien, "Benzodiazepine Use, Abuse, and Dependence"; Golombok, Moodley, and Lader, "Cognitive Impairment in Long-Term Benzodiazepine Users"; Hirschtritt, Olfson, and Korenke, "Balancing the Risks and Benefits of Benzodiazepines."

64. Nicola Simola and Manolo Carta, "Amphetamine Usage, Misuse, and Addiction Processes: An Overview," in *Neuropathology of Drug Addictions and Substance Misuse*, vol. 2, *Stimulants, Club and Dissociative Drugs, Hallucinogens, Steroids, Inhalants and International Aspects*, ed. Victor Preedy (Academic Press, 2016), 14–24; Luise Kazda et al., "Overdiagnosis of Attention-Deficit/Hyperactivity Disorder in Children and Adolescents," *JAMA Network Open* 4, no. 4 (April 12, 2021): e215335.

65. Jorge Vásconez-González et al., "Effects of Smoking Marijuana on the Respiratory System: A Systematic Review," *Substance Abuse* 44, no. 3 (July 1, 2023): 249–260; Marta Di Forti et al., "The Contribution of Cannabis Use to Variation in the Incidence of Psychotic Disorder Across Europe (EU-GEI): A Multicentre Case-Control Study," *Lancet Psychiatry* 6, no. 5 (March 19, 2019): 427–436; National Academies of Sciences, Engineering, and Medicine, *Cannabis Policy Impacts Public Health and Health Equity* (Washington, DC: The National Academies Press, 2024), https://doi.org/10.17226/27766; Carsten Hjorthøj, Christine Merrild Posselt, and Merete Nordentoft, "Development Over Time of the Population-Attributable Risk Fraction for Cannabis Use Disorder in Schizophrenia in Denmark," *JAMA Psychiatry* 78, no. 9 (July 21, 2021): 1013–1019; J. Vaucher et al., "Cannabis Use and Risk of Schizophrenia: A Mendelian Randomization Study," *Molecular Psychiatry* 23, no. 5 (January 24, 2017): 1287–1292.

66. Madeline H. Meier et al., "Persistent Cannabis Users Show Neuropsychological Decline From Childhood to Midlife," *Proceedings of the National Academy of Sciences* 109, no. 40 (August 27, 2012): E2657–2664; Kate Z. Peters, Erik B. Oleson, and Joseph F. Cheer, "A Brain on Cannabinoids: The Role of Dopamine Release in Reward Seeking and Addiction," *Cold Spring Harbor Perspectives in Medicine* 11, no. 1 (January 21, 2020): a039305; David A. Gorelick, "Cannabis-Related Disorders and Toxic Effects," *New England Journal of Medicine* 389, no. 24 (December 13, 2023): 2267–2275.

67. Amy N. Dalton and Stephen A. Spiller, "Too Much of a Good Thing: The Benefits of Implementation Intentions Depend on the Number of Goals," *Journal of Consumer Research* 39, no. 3 (January 26, 2012): 600–614.

68. Chenglong Li et al., "Association of Cumulative Blood Pressure with Cognitive Decline, Dementia, and Mortality," *Journal of the American College of Cardiology* 79, no. 14 (April 1, 2022): 1321–1335.

69. Ehrlich et al., "Addition of Vision Impairment to a Life-Course Model of Potentially Modifiable Dementia Risk Factors in the US"; Lin et al., "Hearing Loss and Cognitive Decline in Older Adults;" Liu Yang et al., "Depression, Depression Treatments, and Risk of Incident Dementia: A Prospective Cohort Study of 354,313 Participants," *Biological Psychiatry* 93, no. 9 (May 1, 2023): 802–809; Zhang et al., "A Meta-Analysis of Cohort Studies."

70. Pedersen and Saltin, "Exercise as Medicine."

71. Wang et al., "A Systematic Review and Meta-Analysis of 90 Cohort Studies of Social Isolation, Loneliness and Mortality."

72. Ellen Meara, Seth Richards, and David M. Cutler, "The Gap Gets Bigger: Changes in Mortality and Life Expectancy, by Education, 1981–2000," *Health Affairs* 27, no. 2 (March 1, 2008): 350–360.

73. Fergus I.M. Craik, Ellen Bialystok, and Morris Freedman, "Delaying the Onset of Alzheimer Disease: Bilingualism as a Form of Cognitive Reserve," *Neurology* 75, no. 19 (November 9, 2010): 1726–1729; Ahmed Arafa et al., "Playing a Musical Instrument and the Risk of

Dementia Among Older Adults: A Systematic Review and Meta-Analysis of Prospective Cohort Studies," *BMC Neurology* 22, no. 1 (October 27, 2022): 395.

74. Lan Anh Nguyen, Karen Murphy, and Glenda Andrews, "Immediate and Long-Term Efficacy of Executive Functions Cognitive Training in Older Adults: A Systematic Review and Meta-Analysis," *Psychological Bulletin* 145, no. 7 (July 1, 2019): 698–733.

75. Sai Tian et al., "Comparison on Cognitive Outcomes of Antidiabetic Agents for Type 2 Diabetes: A Systematic Review and Network Meta-Analysis," *Diabetes/Metabolism Research and Reviews* 39, no. 7 (June 11, 2023): e3673; Bowen Tang et al., "Comparative Effectiveness of Glucagon-like Peptide-1 Agonists, Dipeptidyl Peptidase-4 Inhibitors, and Sulfonylureas on the Risk of Dementia in Older Individuals with Type 2 Diabetes in Sweden: An Emulated Trial Study," *EClinicalMedicine* 73 (June 1, 2024): 102689.

76. Yao Yao et al., "The Effect of China's Clean Air Act on Cognitive Function in Older Adults: A Population-Based, Quasi-Experimental Study," *Lancet Healthy Longevity* 3, no. 2 (February 1, 2022): e98–108.

77. Artitaya Lophatananon et al., "The Association of Herpes Zoster and Influenza Vaccinations with the Risk of Developing Dementia: A Population-Based Cohort Study Within the UK Clinical Practice Research Datalink," *BMC Public Health* 23 (October 2, 2023): 1903; Maxime Taquet et al., "The Recombinant Shingles Vaccine Is Associated with Lower Risk of Dementia," *Nature Medicine* 30, no. 10 (July 25, 2024): 2777–2781; Shah et al., "Herpes Zoster Vaccination and the Risk of Dementia: A Systematic Review and Meta-analysis," *Brain and Behavior* 14, no. 2 (February 1, 2024): e3415; Markus Eyting et al., "A Natural Experiment on the Effect of Herpes Zoster Vaccination on Dementia," *Nature* (April 2, 2025).

78. Sorayya Kheirouri and Mohammad Alizadeh, "MIND Diet and Cognitive Performance in Older Adults: A Systematic Review," *Critical Reviews in Food Science and Nutrition* 62, no. 29 (May 14, 2021): 8059–8077.

79. Mathew J. Reeves and Ann P. Rafferty, "Healthy Lifestyle Characteristics Among Adults in the United States, 2000," *Archives of Internal Medicine* 165, no. 8 (April 25, 2005): 854; Paul D. Loprinzi et al., "Healthy Lifestyle Characteristics and Their Joint Association with Cardiovascular Disease Biomarkers in US Adults," *Mayo Clinic Proceedings* 91, no. 4 (April 1, 2016): 432–442.

EPILOGUE

1. Barron H. Lerner, *One for the Road: Drunk Driving Since 1900* (Baltimore, MD: Johns Hopkins University Press, 2011).

2. WHO, *Global Tuberculosis Report 2023*.

3. Rosling, *Factfulness*, 86–89.

4. Masagus M. Ridhwan et al., "The Effect of Health on Economic Growth: A Meta-Regression Analysis," *Empirical Economics* 63 (April 11, 2022): 3211–3251.

5. Adam Smith, *The Wealth of Nations* (London: W. Strahan and T. Cadell, 1776).

6. Elizabeth A. McGlynn et al., "The Quality of Health Care Delivered to Adults in the United States," *New England Journal of Medicine* 348, no. 26 (June 26, 2003): 2635–2645.

7. Thomas R. Frieden et al., "The Road to Achieving Epidemic-Ready Primary Health Care," *Lancet Public Health* 8, no. 5 (May 1, 2023): e383–390. One good example is Thailand, where successive governments, both military and civilian, protected and expanded primary health care services.

8. Vargas and Muiser, "Promoting Universal Financial Protection"; Kanitsorn Sumriddetchka-jorn et al., "Universal Health Coverage and Primary Care, Thailand," *Bulletin of the World Health Organization* 97, no. 6 (April 1, 2019): 415–422.

9. "The Impacts of Climate Change on Human Health in the United States: A Scientific Assessment," U.S. Global Change Research Program, April 4, 2016, accessed March 8, 2025, https://health2016.globalchange.gov/; Marina Romanello et al., "The 2023 Report of the Lancet Countdown on Health and Climate Change: The Imperative for a Health-Centred Response in a World Facing Irreversible Harms," *Lancet* 402, no. 10419 (December 1, 2023): 2346–2394.

10. "U.S. Construction Costs Dropped for Solar, Wind, and Natural Gas-Fired Generators in 2021," US Energy Information Administration, October 3, 2023, accessed March 8, 2025, https://www.eia.gov/todayinenergy/detail.php?id=60562.

11. "Tracking Clean Energy Progress 2023," International Energy Agency, July 2023, https://www.iea.org/reports/tracking-clean-energy-progress-2023.

12. Martyn P. Chipperfield et al., "Detecting Recovery of the Stratospheric Ozone Layer," *Nature* 549, no. 7671 (September 14, 2017): 211–218.

13. Sierra Club, "Beyond Coal," accessed March 8, 2025, https://coal.sierraclub.org/.

APPENDIX 2

1. Life expectancy gains were calculated using the best available studies, converting all-cause mortality reductions to estimated months of life gained. The estimates take into account baseline life expectancy, age at which the action is likely to be taken, and unhealthy behavior rates. Estimates are not adjusted to account for the potential overlap of health benefits of different actions (e.g., sodium reduction and blood pressure control). Benefits will be higher in higher-risk people and lower in lower-risk people. The populations studied were heterogeneous; the effect on any one individual may differ from these averages. The estimates, although uncertain, give a qualitative sense of the potential relative impact of each action based on evidence available as of early 2025.

2. Richard Doll, et al., "Mortality in Relation to Smoking: 50 Years' Observations on Male British Doctors," *BMJ* 328, no. 7455 (2004): 1519–1527.

3. Prospective Studies Collaboration, "Age-Specific Relevance of Usual Blood Pressure to Vascular Mortality"; Muthiah Vaduganathan et al., "Long-Term Benefit of Intensive Blood Pressure Control on Residual Life Span in the Systolic Blood Pressure Intervention Trial (SPRINT)," *JAMA Cardiology* 5, no. 5 (February 26, 2020): 576–581.

4. Colin Baigent et al., "Efficacy and Safety of More Intensive Lowering of LDL Cholesterol: A Meta-Analysis of Data from 170,000 Participants in 26 Randomised Trials," *Lancet* 376, no. 9753 (November 13, 2010): 1670–1681; Daniel E. Soffer et al., "Role of Apolipoprotein B in the Clinical Management of Cardiovascular Risk in Adults: An Expert Clinical Consensus from the National Lipid Association," *Journal of Clinical Lipidology* 18, no. 5 (2024): e647–4663. Current lipid measurements combine hundreds of different molecules, each of which may have different biological effects; future technologies will enable more precise understanding of cardiovascular risk. In any case, the higher the baseline risk, the longer the extension of healthy life expectancy with lowering of unhealthy lipid levels. People with diabetes benefit substantially from control of blood pressure and lipids to lower levels, and newer anti-diabetic agents, particularly GLP-1 agonists and possibly SGLT2 inhibitors, may reduce dementia.

5. Steven C. Moore et al., "Leisure Time Physical Activity of Moderate to Vigorous Intensity and Mortality: A Large Pooled Cohort Analysis," *PLOS Medicine* 9, no. 11 (November 6, 2012): e1001335. The health benefit may be even larger with higher-intensity, more frequent, or longer workout or with exercise that increases strength through resistance training.

6. Jinhui Zhao et al., "Association Between Daily Alcohol Intake and Risk of All-Cause Mortality: A Systematic Review and Meta-Analyses," *JAMA Network Open* 6, no. 3 (March 31, 2023): e236185.

7. Dariush Mozaffarian et al., "Global Sodium Consumption and Death from Cardiovascular Causes," *New England Journal of Medicine* 371, no. 7 (August 14, 2014): 624–634.

8. Janet S. Choi et al., "Association Between Hearing Aid Use and Mortality in Adults with Hearing Loss in the USA: A Mortality Follow-Up Study of a Cross-Sectional Cohort," *Lancet Healthy Longevity* 5, no. 1 (January 15, 2024): e66–e75.

9. Hamish M.E. Foster et al., "Social Connection and Mortality in UK Biobank: A Prospective Cohort Analysis," *BMC Medicine* 21, 384 (November 10, 2023). Studies suggest even larger increases in longevity; however, there may be unrecognized confounders that account for much of the difference.

10. Qianyi Wang et al., "Impact of Nonoptimal Intakes of Saturated, Polyunsaturated, and Trans Fat on Global Burdens of Coronary Heart Disease," *Journal of the American Heart Association* 5, no. 1 (January 20, 2016): e002891; Yanping Li et al., "Saturated Fats Compared with Unsaturated Fats and Sources of Carbohydrates in Relation to Risk of Coronary Heart Disease: A Prospective Cohort Study," *Journal of the American College of Cardiology* 66, no. 14 (October 6, 2015): 1538–1548. The United States and most of the world have eliminated trans fats from the food supply.

11. Itziar Abete et al., "Association Between Total, Processed, Red, and White Meat Consumption and All-Cause, Cardiovascular, and Cancer Mortality: A Meta-Analysis of Cohort Studies," *British Journal of Nutrition* 112, no. 5 (June 16, 2014): 762–775; Huifeng Zhang et al., "Meat Consumption and Risk of Incident Dementia: Cohort Study of 493,888 UK Biobank Participants," *American Journal of Clinical Nutrition* 114, no. 1 (July 1, 2021): 175–184; Yuhan Li et al., "Long-Term Intake of Red Meat in Relation to Dementia Risk and Cognitive Function in US Adults," *Neurology* 104, no. 3 (February 11, 2025): e210286.

12. Amy Mullee et al., "Association Between Soft Drink Consumption and Mortality in 10 European Countries," *JAMA Internal Medicine* 179, no. 11 (September 3, 2019): 1479–1490.

13. Francesco P. Cappuccio et al., "Sleep Duration and All-Cause Mortality: A Systematic Review and Meta-Analysis of Prospective Studies," *Sleep* 33, no. 5 (May 1, 2010): 585–592.

14. Michael Bretthauer, "Estimated Lifetime Gained with Cancer Screening Tests: A Meta-Analysis of Randomized Clinical Trials," *JAMA Internal Medicine* 183, no. 1 (2023): 19–28.

15. Dan Zhao et al., "Evaluating the Long-Term Health and Economic Impacts of Central Residential Air Filtration for Reducing Premature Mortality Associated with Indoor Fine Particulate Matter (PM2.5) of Outdoor Origin," *International Journal of Environmental Research and Public Health* 12, no. 7 (July 21, 2015): 8448–8479. The benefit will vary based on level of pollution, efficacy of filters, and amount of time exposed at home versus elsewhere.

16. Lophatananon et al., "The Association of Herpes Zoster and Influenza Vaccinations"; Taquet et al., "The Recombinant Shingles Vaccine"; Shah et al., "Herpes Zoster Vaccination and the Risk of Dementia"; Eyting et al., "A Natural Experiment on the Effect of Herpes Zoster Vaccination on Dementia."

17. Lara M. Wittine et al., "Mortality Among Veterans Following Traumatic Brain Injury: A Veterans Administration Traumatic Brain Injury Model System Study," *Journal of Neurotrauma* 42, no. 7–8 (April 17, 2025): 745–757.

18. Among people with depression, the longevity benefits of effective treatment may be substantial. Helen-Maria Vasiliadis et al., "Minimally Adequate Treatment for Depression and Anxiety Associated with Mortality in Primary Care Older Adults," *Canadian Journal of Psychiatry* 67, no. 9 (March 7, 2022): 669–678.

19. Craik, Bialystok, and Freedman, "Delaying the Onset of Alzheimer Disease"; Arafa et al., "Playing a Musical Instrument and the Risk of Dementia Among Older Adults"; B Løkken, "Are Playing Instruments, Singing or Creating Theatre Good for Health? Associations with Self-Related Health and All-Cause Mortality in the HUNT3 Study (2006–08), Norway," *European Journal of Public Health* 27, suppl. 3 (November 2017): ckx187.543 (abstract).

Related Reading

Barry, John M. *The Great Influenza: The Story of the Deadliest Pandemic in History*. New York: Penguin Books, 2016.

Brandt, Allan M. *The Cigarette Century: The Rise, Fall, and Deadly Persistence of the Product That Defined America*. New York: Basic Books, 2007.

Crofton, John. *Tobacco: A Global Threat*. New York: Macmillan, 2002.

Foege, William H. *The Fears of the Rich, the Needs of the Poor: My Years at the CDC*. Baltimore, MD: Johns Hopkins University Press, 2018.

Foege, William H. *House on Fire: The Fight to Eradicate Smallpox*. Berkeley: University of California Press, 2011.

Foege, William H. *The Task Force for Child Survival: Secrets of Successful Coalitions*. Baltimore, MD: Johns Hopkins University Press, 2018.

Johnson, Steven. *The Ghost Map: The Story of London's Most Terrifying Epidemic—and How It Changed Science, Cities, and the Modern World*. New York: Riverhead Books, 2006.

Katz, Rebecca, and Mackenzie S. Moore. *The Outbreak Atlas*. Nashville, TN: Vanderbilt University Press, 2024.

Lerner, Barron H. *One for the Road: Drunk Driving Since 1900*. Baltimore, MD: Johns Hopkins University Press, 2011.

Ryan, Frank. *The Forgotten Plague: How the Battle Against Tuberculosis Was Won—and Lost*. Boston: Little, Brown, 1993.

Oshinsky, David M. *Polio: An American Story*. New York: Oxford University Press, 2005.

Rose, Geoffrey. *The Strategy of Preventive Medicine*. New York: Oxford University Press, 1992.

Rosling, Hans, with Ola Rosling and Anna Rosling Rönnlund. *Factfulness: Ten Reasons We're Wrong About the World—and Why Things Are Better Than You Think*. New York: Flatiron Books, 2018.

Shilts, Randy. *And the Band Played On: Politics, People, and the AIDS Epidemic*. New York: St. Martin's Press, 1987.

Index

Accountable Care Organizations, 74

Addams, Jane, 12

Advocacy, 110, 136–137

Aedes aegypti mosquito, 70–71

Affordable Care Act, 22

Ahlers, Charles, 136

Alcohol, 45, 156, 180, 186, 192, 205–207

Algorithms, simplicity in, 98–99

American Beverage Association, 131–132

American Public Health Association, 61

Angel (tuberculosis patient), 148–149, 150, 151

Anthony, Susan B., 12

Aravind Eye Care System, 94

Ardern, Jacinda, 118–119

Australia, 117–118

Austria, ban on indoor lead paint, 14

Azar, Alex, 80

Bacteriophages, 209n1

Barbot, Oxiris, 105, 107

Battle of Quebec, 59

Beal, Susan, 42

Belgium, ban on indoor lead paint, 14

Bell, Eleanor, xii, 5

Beyond Coal campaign, 194

Biases
  negativity, 225n24
  normalcy, 32, 157, 162
  optimism, 71–72

Biden, Joseph, 122, 143

Biggs, Hermann, 9, 143

Bihar, India, 67

Bill and Melinda Gates Foundation, 60

Binge drinking, 186, 207, 247n60

Birx, Deborah, 80, 103

Blood pressure. *See* Hypertension

Bloomberg Initiative to Reduce Tobacco Use, 109

Bloomberg, Mike, xiv, 17, 52, 145, 148, 189, 236n14
  and MPOWER technical package, 52, 109
  smokers and smoking ban, 28, 29, 133, 137–139
  and tax on sugar-sweetened beverages (soda tax), 131–132, 156–157
  and tobacco tax, 18

Bloomberg Philanthropies, 194

Bloomberg School of Public Health (Johns Hopkins University), 90

Brazil, 165

Breast cancer, 46–47

BREATHE (Bar and Restaurant Employees Advocating Together for a Healthy Environment), 138

Breathing exercises, and lower blood pressure, 244n29

Breed, London, 104–105

Broad Street pump, 168

Brudney, Karen, xi, xii, xv, xvi, xvii, 3, 5, 9, 82–83, 86–87, 149, 162–163, 168
and Styblo, 96
Burden × Amenability, 46–47, 52, 55, 60, 108, 166–167, 179, 181
Burial practices, 210n5
Bush, George W., 30, 108–109
Butts, Calvin, 138

Carter, Jimmy, 93
Carter Center, 60, 93
Cassandra (mythical priestess), xiii
Cassandra curse, xiii, 6
drivers of, 21–32, 33–34, 161–162, 202
Centers for Disease Control and Prevention (CDC), xi, xii, 4, 5, 80, 164
annual summary, 21
budget, 144–145
and coronavirus, 54
coronavirus testing error, 229n9
and COVID (see COVID-19)
and Ebola in West African countries, 35, 36, 37, 77–78, 92, 102
Epidemic Intelligence Service, 87, 89, 105, 112–113, 150, 155
laboratories, 145
and Marburg virus infection, 37–38
messaging, 117
and Million Hearts initiative, 22–23
and PFAS levels, 16
and public health advisors, 85
recommendation of hard-hitting anti-tobacco advertising, 18
team building, 83
Tips from Former Smokers campaign, 123, 233n16
tobacco laboratory, 25–26
trust in, 122
Centers for Medicare and Medicaid Services, 22
Checklist Manifesto: How to Get Things Right, The (Gawande), 86

Cherner, Joe, 137–139
China, 103, 164
Guangdong Province, 166
Chinatown (New York City), 40, 166
Cholesterol. *See* Lipids
Cleveland Clinic, 74
Clinton, Bill, 127
Coca-Cola, 132–134, 136
Cohort monitoring, to track progress, 95–97
Collins, Francis, 143
Commercial interests, 140–143
Communication, 115–116
audience, 124–125
failure, 118–121
and messenger, 121–124
and miscommunication, 125–126
the right message, 117–118
and trust, 126–129
Comstock, George, 44
Conde, Alpha, 150
Confidentiality, public health, 211n11
Contagion (movie), 39
Copenhagen, 195
Corruption, 90–92, 227n15
Coronavirus Task Force, 80
Costa Rica, 32, 74, 193
Covey, Stephen, 81
COVID-19, 79–80, 103–107, 161–163
and CDC funding, 145, 146
and disease surveillance, 10
and masking, 127–128, 151, 152, 153
and messaging, 119–120, 122
in New York City, 103–106
outbreak on Diamond Princess cruise ship, 54
Partnership for Evidence-Based Response to COVID, 124
in San Francisco, 104–105
spreading widely, 53–54
tracking with R_0, 39–40
vaccine, mask, and other mandates, 151–154

Crofton, John, 191–192, 196
Cuba, 74
Cuomo, Andrew, 106
Czech Republic, 147

Dan (author's uncle), 175, 182, 187
"Dead Lenny's Title," 88–89, 162
de Blasio, Bill, 104–105, 107
Debs, Eugene V., 12, 212n20
Dementia, 187–189, 205–208, 244n29
Dewey, John, 12
Diamond Princess cruise ship, outbreak of
    COVID on, 54
Dinkins, David, 136
DOTS, 51–52
Douglas, Tennessee, 115–116, 124, 125, 171
Drucker, Peter, 29–29
Drugs for Neglected Diseases initiative
    (DNDi), 94
Duncan, Thomas Eric, 36, 38–39, 41
Dunkin' Donuts, 234n19

Early Head Start, 144
Ebola, in West African countries, 6–8, 35–41,
    77–79, 92–93, 101–102, 112–114, 123,
    150–151, 210n4, 210n5
Economic incentives, and the health care
    system, 24–25, 141, 202
Eisenhower, Dwight, 81, 98
Endocrine disruptors, 16
Epidemics That Didn't Happen (report), 62
Estonia, 91
Evelyn (author's grandmother), 187–188
Evidence. *See* Randomized controlled trial
    (RCT)
Evidence-based programs, 42. *See also*
    Randomized controlled trial (RCT)

False alarms, 30–31, 33, 34, 162, 202
Farr, William, 10
Fauci, Tony, 80, 103
Feynman, Richard, 15

Fink, Shea, 133
Finland, 195
Foege, Bill, 59–60, 77, 135
France, ban on indoor lead paint, 14
Frankfurter, Felix, 12
Franklin, Benjamin, 59, 125–126
Free will, myth of unfettered, 21, 25–28, 33,
    162, 202
Freud, Sigmund, 90

Gasoline, and lead poisoning, 12–15, 213n26
Gates Foundation, 60
Gawande, Atul, 86
Gaynor, Pete, 80
Geisinger, 74, 183
Giuliani, Rudy, 136
Gonorrhea, 62
Graunt, John, 8–9, 10, 21, 194
Great Society, 116
Guangdong Province, China, 166
Gueye, Abdou Salam, 150
Guinea, 6, 35, 77, 102, 150

Hall, Terrie, 123
Hamburg, Margaret "Peggy," 87
Hamilton, Alice, 12–15, 16, 23, 25, 29, 141,
    212n24, 213n26
Hamilton, Edith, 12
Harlem (New York City), 145
Harlem Hospital, 94
Health Defense Operations, 146
Health impact pyramid, 47–50
HEARTS (technical package), 52–53, 93,
    98–100, 169–172
Henderson, Yandell, 14
HEPA filters, 177
Hepatitis, 62, 187
Hiring, 86–90
HIV, xi, xiv, 3, 4, 5, 10, 53, 62, 117, 149
    and tuberculosis, 218n4
H1N1 influenza, 146
Hoover, Margaret, 103

House on Fire (Foege), 60
Hull House Settlement (Chicago), 12
Humility, 53–55
Hyperbolic discounting, 21, 31–32, 33, 34, 61, 138, 157, 162, 178, 202
Hypertension, xv, 98, 100, 175–176, 183
  Black Americans and, 10
  and Burden × Amenability calculation, 49–50, 52
  control rate, 24, 53
  diagnosis of, 98
  information systems for, 99–100
  monitoring treatment program progress, 99–100
  as longer-term risk, 31
  mass screening for, ineffectiveness of, 72, 225n25
  and matrix to manage public health time and resources, 81–83, 226–227n4
  and other health risks, 46–47, 112
  as a pandemic that can be controlled, 169–172
  and prioritization, 81, 226–227n4
  prevention of, 172, 240–241n30
  risk assessment, inadvisability of performing prior to starting treatment, 228n2
  and socioeconomic status, 221n34
  technical package to control (HEARTS), 52–53, 93, 98–100, 169–172
  treatment of, 46–47, 50, 98–100, 180, 183, 188, 205, 207
  universal measurement of blood pressure, 225n25
Hypertension treatment algorithm, 99–100, 226–227n4

Incident management and incident management systems, 78–81
  and COVID, 106, 122
India, 63–70, 94, 135
Information systems, simplicity in, 99–100
Inouye, Daniel, 144

Institutions, principles for success, 84–86
Intermountain Health, 74
Italy, 103

Japan, 128
Johns Hopkins University, Bloomberg School of Public Health, 90
Jorge (patient with hemophilia), 122–123
Jungle, The (Sinclair), 12

Kaiser Permanente, 25, 74, 142, 170, 183
Kappa, 39–41
Keynes, John Maynard, 127
Khan Academy, 195
Khatri, G. R., 66, 67–69, 90–91, 70, 134–135
King, Martin Luther, Jr., 101
Kushner, Jared, 80

Lagos, Nigeria, 35, 77–79, 102
Lassa fever, 166
Layton, Marci, 105–107
Lead paint, in the United States, 14–15
Lead poisoning, 10–15, 212n24
League of Nations, 14
Leiter, Al, 138
Lenny (New York City government worker), 88–89
Liberia, 6, 35, 37, 77, 101, 102
Lindblade, Kim, 113
Lipids, 176, 180, 205, 207, 241n5, 251n4
Liu, Joanne, 92–93
Longevity, and stress, 246n54
LPG (liquefied petroleum gas), 108, 231n27
Luelmo, Fabio, 68, 97
Luntz, Frank, 117
Luwero, Uganda, 102

Madison Square Garden, 105
Madonia, Peter, 40, 139
Mahoney, Frank, 101–102, 113
Malaria, 11, 71, 194
Marburg virus, 37–38, 165, 199

Masks, 127–128, 237n26
  and mandates, 151–153
Matrix to manage public health time and
    resources, 81–83
Mauthausen-Gusen concentration camp
    (Austria), 39
Mayo Clinic, 74
McDonald's, 234n19
Mead, Margaret, 136
Médecins Sans Frontières (MSF), 92–93, 94
Medicare, 32, 171
Medication donation programs, 143, 236n11
Meltzer, Martin, 6–7, 19, 210n4
Messonnier, Nancy, 54, 106, 120
Microbiome, 177
Million Hearts initiative, 22–24, 25, 27, 170
Mississippi Delta, viii
Minnesota, 37
Miscommunication, 125–126. *See also*
    Communication
Mitchell, Edwin, 41–42
Monrovia, Liberia, 36, 92, 101
Mostashari, Farzad, 17–18, 103, 106, 214n46
Mother Jones, 12
Mountin, Joseph, 85
MPOWER (technical package), 52, 109–110
Myers, Matt, 137

Nanny state critique, 154–157
National Institute of Allergy and Infectious
    Diseases, 80
National Institutes of Health, 143, 164
*Natural and Political Observations Made upon
    the Bills of Mortality* (Graunt), 8–9
Negativity bias, 225n24
New Deal, farming programs, 115
New Delhi, 66, 134, 191
New England Journal of Medicine, 131
New York City, 17–19, 27, 28–29, 30, 40,
    124, 149, 167, 168
  Board of Health, xii, 124
  Chinatown, 166

City Council, 18, 137, 138, 139
  clean water in, 132–133
  community health survey, 86
  COVID in, 103–106
  government job titles, 88–89
  Health Code, xii
  Health Department, xi, xii, 4, 61, 87, 118,
    143
  smoking and tobacco in, 176, 137–138,
    147
  and tuberculosis, 36, 63, 82–84, 94–97,
    101, 162
New York Coalition to Eliminate
    Tuberculosis, 136
New York State, health department, 143
New York State Medical Society, 155
New York Times (newspaper), 35
New Zealand, 41–43, 118–120
Nichol, Stuart, 38, 77
Nigeria, 10–12, 59, 77–79
Nongovernmental organizations, 92–94
Normalcy bias, 32, 157, 162
Nurse-Family Partnership (NFP), 110–112
Nwigwe, Christian, 122–123

Obama, Barack, xiv, 35, 101–102
Olds, David, 110–112
Operation Warp Speed, 107
Optimism
  irrational, 69–70
  maintaining, 72–74
  misplaced, 70–72
  power of, 67–69
Optimism bias, 71–72
"Ounces of Prevention—the Public Policy
    Case for Taxes on Sugared Beverages"
    (Brownell and Frieden), 131

Pandemics. *See also specific pandemics, e.g.*
    COVID-19
  finding faster, 167–168
  preventing, 161–167

Pandemics (cont.)
stopping cholera, a current pandemic, 168–169
stopping hypertension, the world's deadliest pandemic, 169–172
and surveillance, 167–168
Partnership for Evidence-Based Response to COVID, 124–125
Patterson, David, 131
Paxlovid, 120
Payne-Yehuda, Martinah, 137–138
Pence, Mike, 80
PepsiCo, 132–134, 136
Peru, 168
Pet ownership, and exercise, 242n16
Pew Research Center, 126–127
PFAS (per- and polyfluoroalkyl substances), 16, 177
Pham, Nina, 36
Philadelphia, 157
Philip Morris, 27
Pirkle, Jim, 25–27
President's Emergency Plan for AIDS Relief (PEPFAR), 108–109, 111
Prevention and Public Health Fund, 55–56
Prevention paradox, 21–24, 28, 33, 132, 162, 172, 178, 202, 231n17
Primary health care, 168, 171, 179, 183
and optimism, 73–74
reasons for lack of, 32–34, 142
See/Believe/Formula to improve, 192–194
Prioritization, 81–82
Program performance, tracking, 17–19 Project BioWatch, 30
Public Broadcasting System (PBS), 103
Public health, 3, 17, 28, 45–46, 48–50, 55–56, 78, 82, 106–107, 133, 139, 161–163, 168, 196
and commercial interests, 140–143
and dementia, 187–189
formula for, 175–177
funding, 143–148

and a healthy future, 177–187
law, 148–151
mandates, 151–154
and "nanny state" critique, 154–157
past progress in, 61–63
and personal politics, 189–190
surveillance and, 8–10, 19, 60, 86, 157
Public health policies, 109–110, 131–132, 156–157, 171, 189–190. *See also* Commercial interests
and advocacy and partnerships, 136–137
and deciders and influencers, 134–136
and pragmatism, and timing, 137–140
and winners and losers, 132–134
Purchasing and contracting processes, 227n15
Python Cave, 37

Queen Elizabeth Park, Uganda, 37

R_0, 39–40, 218n4, 218–219n6
Randomized controlled trial (RCT), 42–46
Rapid Isolation and Treatment of Ebola (RITE), 113
Red meat consumption, reducing 243n21
REPLACE (technical package), 52
Reproduction number (R_0), 39–40
limitations of, 218–219n6
Resolve to Save Lives, xiv, 52, 62, 80–81, 93, 98, 106
Partnership for Evidence-Based Response to COVID, 124–125
Revolutionary War, 59
Risk analysis, 228n2
Riva-Rocci, Scipione, 176, 241n1
Roosevelt, Eleanor, 115
Rose, Geoffrey, 23, 28, 148
Rosling, Hans, 47, 61, 73, 113
Rule of halves, 32

Salinas, Louis, 83–84, 85
San Francisco, COVID in, 104–105

SARS-1, 166
Saunas, 244n29
Sawyer, Patrick, 77–78
Sbarbaro, John, 191
Scale and scaling, 107–110, 112–114
    scalability, 110–112
Seattle, 103
See/Believe/Create formula, xv, 74, 81, 91,
    94, 97, 114, 118, 137, 157, 161, 175,
    194, 195, 203
Senate Appropriations Committee, 144
7-1-7, target for rapid detection, reporting,
    and response to health threats, 107, 167
Shakespeare, William, 187
Sierra Leone, 6, 35, 77, 102, 151, 194, 195
Simple, application for digital monitoring of
    hypertension and diabetes, 100
Simplicity and simplification, 95–101,
    112–114
Sinclair, Upton, 12
Singapore, 91
Single overriding communication objective
    (SOCO), 118
Skyler, Ed, 133
Slip-Slop-Slap campaign, 118
Smallpox, eradication, 59–60, 61, 125–126,
    135, 164, 224n4, 224n5
Smith, Adam, 192
Smoking and smokers, in New York City,
    176
Snow, John, 168
Social isolation, 244n29
Social norms, 21, 28–30, 33, 34, 162, 178,
    202
Soda tax, 131–132, 136, 155–157
Soper, Fred, 70–71
South Bronx (New York City), 145
South Korea, 128
Soviet Union, 164
Speed, 101–103, 112–114
Sri Lanka, 74
Standard Oil Company (New Jersey), 13–14

Stark, Martha, 147
Staten Island (New York City), 28
St. Clare's Hospital, 5
Steps to a long, healthy life, 205–208, 250n1,
    251n4, 251n10, 252n15, 252n18
    and alcohol consumption, 45, 180, 186,
        188, 205, 207
    and brain injury, 188, 208
    and cancer screening, 208
    and depression, 180, 188, 208, 252n18
    and hearing, 180, 188, 207
    and HEPA filters, 208
    and lipids, 176, 180, 205, 207, 241n5,
        251n4
    and physical activity, 180, 184, 206–207,
        251n5
    and playing a musical instrument, 180,
        189, 208
    and potassium consumption, 172, 180,
        184, 207, 242–243n18
    and processed meats, 207, 243n21
    and sleep, 180, 185, 206, 208
    and social connections, 180, 207, 251n9
    and sodium consumption, 45, 49, 172, 180,
        184, 207, 242–243n18
    and speaking a second language or playing a
        musical instrument, 180, 208
    and stress, 246n54
    and sugary beverages, 180, 208
    and tobacco use, 180, 185, 188, 205, 207
    and vaccination, 208
    and vision, 180, 188, 207
Strep throat, 62
Stress, and longevity, 246n54
Styblo, Karel, xvi, 39–40, 51–52, 66, 95, 100,
    110, 111, 134, 149, 191
    and Brudney, 96–97
    technical package for tuberculosis control,
        51–52, 83, 93, 95, 162
Sudden infant death syndrome (SIDS), 41,
    42
Superspreading, 41, 219n9, 219n10

Surveillance, 4, 5, 60, 86, 157
  and health data, 8–10, 211n13
  and pollution in New York City air,
    236n14
  syndromic, 103
Syndromic surveillance, 103

Tanzania, 40
Teams, 82–84
Technical packages, 50–53
Technical rigor, 35–36, 38–41, 179, 203. *See
  also* Burden × Amenability, Health impact
  pyramid, and Technical packages
  and humility, 53–55
  and J-shaped statistical relationships, 44–46
  and program-based evidence,
    41–44Thailand, 32, 74, 193
"There's Plenty of Room at the Bottom"
  (Feynman), 15
Tips from Former Smokers campaign (CDC),
    123, 233n16
Tobacco use, 109–110, 111, 112, 133, 141,
    185–186, 188–189, 192
  and hard-hitting advertising, 123, 233n16
  in Million Hearts initiative, 22–24
  and taxation, 146–148
  and tobacco industry, 25–27
  and MPOWER technical package, 52
  and smoke-free laws, 135–139
  in New York City, 16–19
Tonkin, Shirley, 42
Toxins, invisible, 15–16
Trans fats, ban in New York City, 123–124,
    234n19
Transmission risk, 218–219n6
Transparency International, 92
Trump, Donald, 54, 80, 105, 106, 118–122,
    127
Tuberculosis
  drug-resistant, xi, xii, xv, xvi, xvii, 3–5, 9,
    82–83, 86–87, 149, 162–163, 168
  and HIV, 218n4

leading cause of death from infectious
    disease, 222–223n46
  reduction in deaths from, 51–52
Tufte, Edward, 18
Twain, Mark, 148, 189

Uganda, 37, 102, 106–107
United Kingdom, 53, 101, 164, 193
United States
  Congress, 27, 55, 144, 145
  Department of Health and Human Services,
    22–23, 55, 80
  Federal Communications Commission
    (FCC), 27
  Federal Emergency Management Agency
    (FEMA), 80
  Food and Drug Administration (FDA),
    22–23, 171
  Government Accountability Office, 30
  Office of Management and Budget, 144,
    145–146
  White House, 22, 55
United States Chamber of Commerce, 136
University of Auckland School of Medicine,
    41
Uruguay, 135

Vaccine mandates, COVID-19, 153–154
Vaishali, Bihar, 64–65
Vajpayee, Atal, 134
Varmus, Harold, 137
Vázquez, Tabaré, 135
Vermont, 137
Vinson, Amber, 36
Vir, Gautam, 64–65, 67
Virchow, Rudolph, 50
Vitruvius, 11

Washington, DC, 30
Washington, George, 59
West African countries, Ebola in, 35, 36, 37,
    77–78, 92, 102

West Bengal, 17, 22, 55, 90–91

Wet markets, 166

White, Ryan, 117

WHO (World Health Organization), 35, 51–
52, 63–64, 68, 97, 98

Wilson, James Q., 84, 136

Winslet, Kate, 39

Winslow, C.-E. A., 61

World Bank, 63, 191

World Health Organization (WHO), 35, 51–
52, 63–64, 68, 97, 98

World Summit for Children (1980), 109

Zika emergency, 146